John P.

Pelican Books
Man, Medicine and En

René Dubos was born in Saint-Brice, France, in
1901, and attended the Institut National
Agronomique in Paris. In 1924 he went to the
United States and he became a U.S. citizen in
1938. He was awarded a Ph.D. by Rutgers
University in 1927 and has been a faculty member
of the Rockefeller University since that time,
except for the period 1942–4, when he was
George Fabyan Professor of Comparative
Pathology and Tropical Medicine at Harvard
University Medical School.

His interest in the effects of the total environment
has led him increasingly into sociomedical
problems. One result is his demonstration that
early environmental influences can have lasting
effects on the anatomical, physiological and
behavioural characteristics of adult animals
and man.

Dr Dubos has been an editor of the *Journal of
Experimental Medicine* since 1946, and has
written many books, his most recent, besides
the present volume, being: *Mirage of Health,
The Torch of Life, Man Adapting, So Human
an Animal* (which won the Pulitzer Prize in
1969) and *Reason Awake! Science for Man.* He
is a member of the National Academy of
Sciences and the American Philosophical Society,
and has received honorary degrees from twenty-
three American and other universities, as well
as many American and international awards.

René Dubos

Man, Medicine and Environment

Penguin Books

Penguin Books Ltd, Harmondsworth,
Middlesex, England
Penguin Books Australia Ltd, Ringwood,
Victoria, Australia

First published in the U.S.A. 1968
Published in Great Britain by The Pall Mall Press 1968
Published in Pelican Books 1970

Man, Medicine and Environment is a *Britannica
Perspective* prepared to commemorate the
two hundredth anniversary of
Encyclopaedia Britannica

Made and printed in Great Britain
by C. Nicholls & Company Ltd
Set in Linotype Times

Contents

1 The Living World

The Great Chain of Being

All men are aware of their kinship to animals. Irrespective of their religious or philosophical allegiance, and whatever the sophistication of their scientific knowledge, they perceive in their minds and feel in their hearts the deep philosophical significance of St Francis of Assisi's love for his brothers, the beasts, and of Albert Schweitzer's reverence for life. Indeed, most modern men have come to accept, or at least to tolerate, the concept that all living things have evolved one from the other and are therefore biologically related. Few today take offence at the thought, so disturbing a century ago, that man himself has emerged from a line of descent that began with microbial life, a line common to all plant and animal species.

Widespread acceptance of the evolutionary doctrine is, of course, very recent. It dates from the writings of Charles Darwin, A. R. Wallace and their followers during the second half of the nineteenth century. But the idea that all living things are related was implicit in many ancient religious and philosophical doctrines. Indeed, one may wonder whether this unitarian view of life is not coeval with *Homo sapiens*.

In his learned book, *The Great Chain of Being*, the philosopher Arthur O. Lovejoy has richly illustrated the countless imaginative efforts of men in past civilizations to account for the order that seems to prevail in nature over the arrangement of living things. Size and shape, anatomical structure, physiological properties, preferred habitats and behavioural patterns are among the many characteristics that differentiate the various forms of life and make them appear to constitute well-defined and apparently unchangeable entities. Despite the testimony of the senses that no two creatures are exactly alike, the human mind has made repeated efforts throughout history to classify plants and animals according to a progressive order of complexity and excellence. Naturalists and philosophers have long believed that the various forms of life constitute an orderly chain of many links, each link increasing in complexity from the chain's beginning to its end.

Expressions such as *scala naturae*, or the 'ladder of life', are used frequently throughout ancient literature to symbolize the belief that a majestic hierarchical order prevails over all creation. According to this view, the hierarchy extends from inanimate matter through every possible grade of living existence, culminating in man and reaching toward God. Aristotle stated two thousand years ago that nature 'passes so gradually from inanimate matter to the animate world that their continuity renders the boundary between them indistinguishable; and there is a middle kind that belongs to both orders. For plants come immediately after inanimate things ... and the transition from plants to animals is continuous . . .' Whether life really is continuous with inanimate matter and whether living organisms possess some special attribute not identifiable with known physico-chemical forces are still matters of debate. There is no doubt, in any case, that all living forms have many characteristics in common. Hence the conclusion, supported by fossil evidence, that they all derive from a common origin.

Aristotle himself, and most naturalists and philosophers after him, realized that a creature that appears superior to another with regard to one kind of character may be inferior to it in other regards. They knew, furthermore, that the characteristics of one class of organisms usually shade off into those of another class, and that sharp distinctions between them are in reality artificial. It was eventually recognized that living things can be classified according to many different, so-called natural, systems depending upon the criteria selected by the classifier. For all these reasons many sceptics came to believe that the apparent hierarchical order among living things is an invention of the human mind that has little bearing on the natural state of affairs. Yet the faith remained widespread that living things, especially animals, can be arranged in a single, graded *scala naturae* according to their relative degrees of 'perfection', with man, as the probable image of God, at the top.

One of the consequences of the theory that man – especially the white man – occupies the highest position on the ladder of life was the belief that other living things had been created for his sake. This belief prevailed among medieval schoolmen and was accepted by Francis Bacon: 'Man, if we look to final causes, may be regarded as the centre of the world; insomuch that if man were taken away from the world, the rest would seem to be all astray, without aim or purpose ... and leading to nothing.' The same view was expressed as late as 1784 by Bernardin de Saint-Pierre in his *Études de la nature*: 'The Creator has aimed ... only at the happiness of man. All the laws of nature are designed to serve our needs.' This phrase sounds scientifically naïve today, but there is no doubt that its spirit still governs the behaviour of many men. Descartes and Leibniz rejected on theoretical grounds all attempts at explanation of the universe based on such anthropocentric teleology and philosophy. But public attitude continued to regard man as the focus of creation and its *raison d'être* until evolutionary theories gained general acceptance. The theory of evolution provided a new and plausible dogma to account for the phenomena so long symbolized by the concept of the Great Chain of Being.

Most laymen, as well as theologians, now believe with scientists that life on earth began at least two to three billion years ago; that all its known living forms evolved one from the other through mutation and selection; and that mankind is but the most advanced manifestation of the gradual unfolding of life's potentialities. In the light of the theory of evolution, the interrelation of all living things and the possibility of arranging them according to hierarchical orders are the consequences of a continuous process. Evolutionary development results in the progressive emergence of organisms endowed with greater and greater complexity. Higher animals, reaching their apex in man, are the most complex living things with regard to genetic constitution, behaviour and social organization. Scientific knowledge has thus confirmed the ancient view based on common sense and experience, that man occupies the highest position on the ladder of life. But this is not saying that all creation has been organized for his benefit.

The Web of Life

The theory of progressive change through organic evolution emerged from the vision and dedicated labour of two of the gentlest heroes of science, A. R. Wallace and Charles Darwin. Ironically enough, several nineteenth-century economists and sociologists found in the writing of these guileless and disinterested naturalists a scientific excuse for the harsh policies and bloodcurdling slogans of the Victorian era.

Herbert Spencer and the social Darwinists saw in the theory of evolution a mechanism – supposedly ethical because it was presumed to be based on natural laws – that accounted for the survival of the fittest. In their view, this mechanism explained and justified continued prosperity for the upper social classes. The weeding out of the weak members of animal populations in nature appeared to some Victorians a sufficient excuse for imperialism, sweatshops, child labour and slums.

The social Darwinists held that political and economic progress was best served by applying to human affairs the competitive and destructive practices they assumed to constitute the law of the jungle. This simplistic approach had no scientific justification. Darwin himself rejected the view that organic evolution based on selection of the most vigorous forms depended exclusively on competitive and destructive practices in nature. He had clearly stated that 'in numberless animal societies, struggle is replaced by cooperation'. Thomas H. Huxley, the most ardent and articulate apostle of Darwin during the Victorian era, was much disturbed by the attempts of social Darwinists to apply evolutionary doctrines directly to the political and ethical problems of mankind. In his famous Romanes lecture, delivered in 1893, he acknowledged that 'the animal world is on about the same level as a gladiator show. . . . The strongest, the swiftest, and cunningest live to fight another day . . . no quarter is given.' But as a moralist, he rejected the assumption that this 'gladiatorial theory of existence' was applicable to mankind. While he believed that man had evolved from the beast, he held that the rules of human conduct were different from those of animal behaviour, a dichotomy of view which has not yet been entirely resolved.

The Russian social critic Prince Kropotkin, going even further than Darwin and Huxley, denied that the law of the jungle necessarily implies competitive struggle. During his travels in Siberia and Manchuria, Kropotkin had observed the frequent occurrence of cooperative endeavours in the animal world; moreover, his study of past human institutions had convinced him that a desire for cooperation was natural to man. The popularity of his book *Mutual Aid, a Factor of Evolution*, published at the turn of this century, indicated that social Darwinism was then becoming ethically unacceptable.

It may be permissible at this point to open a parenthesis and consider a few facts that throw a curious light on the interplay between social attitudes and scientific doctrines. In the middle of the nineteenth century, biological study was characterized by emphasis on the competitive aspects of life, with general neglect of the phenomena of cooperation in the animal kingdom. Tennyson reflected this attitude when he wrote of 'Nature, red in tooth and claw'. There is no doubt that tooth-and-claw ethics suited the *laisser faire* economics and imperialistic policies of the Victorian era; to some extent, such an attitude was compatible also with the extreme formula of Marxism in its early aggressive phase. In contrast, scientific interest in the cooperative aspects of animal life increased in the Western world precisely at the time when social mores began to condemn imperialism and social injustice. Peaceful coexistence among living things is now becoming an increasingly fashionable aspect of studies devoted to animal behaviour, just as it has become a doctrine in international relations, even though it is frequently violated in practice.

Scientists might like to believe that the change from tooth-and-claw ethics to social liberalism is a consequence of greater biological knowledge, but there is no basis for this flattering assumption. Nature and the interplay between living organisms have not changed in the past hundred years. In particular, the various forms of cooperative activity in the animal kingdom were as readily accessible for observation and study to Victorian naturalists as they are now to modern biologists. It is probable that the scientific evidence for a liberal social policy as against nineteenth-century social Darwinism does not come from a reassessment of old biological information, but rather from the search for new kinds of information. Scientists are in general remarkably objective in reporting what they observe and measure, but the selection of their objects of study is profoundly influenced by the social environment in which they work and by the spirit of the age. In the mood of the present day, we shall present here evidence that mutual cooperation prevails in the world of nature a cooperation of the kind we like to believe could prevail in the world of men.

Idealistic as he was, Prince Kropotkin did not assume that the many examples of mutual aid he had seen among wild animals resulted from a cooperative spirit based on sentiment. He traced it rather to an instinct for self-preservation, observing that species and individual organisms have a better chance to survive when they cooperate than when they engage in destructive competition. Given the multifarious environmental threats that all creatures have to overcome, peaceful coexistence, Kropotkin believed, was the better part of biological wisdom.

While to devour was long regarded as the only alternative to being devoured, many precise observations reveal that this oversimplified formula explains only a limited aspect of the interplay between living things. It is true that practically all living organisms eventually serve as food for others and that the chain which binds all forms of life is in practice made up of dead bodies. It is equally true, however, that, under natural conditions, the various species that have long coexisted in a given area attain an equilibrium. The most impressive aspect of the law of the jungle is not ruthless competition and destruction, but rather interdependence and coexistence.

Everywhere in nature life is a collective enterprise. All organisms, primitive or complex, naturally spend much of their lives in the company of their own kind; but in addition, and more interestingly, they always occur in intimate and lasting associations with other forms of life not genetically related to them. In fact, most living things, unless cared for by man, soon die of disease or starvation when they are separated from the other species with which they are associated in nature.

While it would be out of place and quite impossible to list here the many different kinds of biological partnerships that have been recognized and studied, it is important to emphasize that such associations occur throughout the living world and involve animals, plants and microbes in almost every imaginable kind of combination. Indeed, many types of organisms long thought to constitute well-defined biological species turn out in reality to be two or more different species. Genetically unrelated, these organisms are so intimately associated and so interdependent that it is commonly difficult to separate one from the other. The word 'symbiosis' was invented approximately one century ago to designate such biological associations mutually advantageous to the associated partners.

Certain groups of biologists have abandoned the original definition of symbiosis and apply the word to any regular association between two different species, whether it involves beneficial mutualism or parasitism resulting in disease and even death. While this definition is consonant with the etymology of the word symbiosis (living together), it is so broad as to be useless. Probably for this reason it is given low priority in most encyclopedias and dictionaries. As used in this book, symbiosis refers to biological associations in which each organism contributes to the survival and welfare of its partner. Recent discoveries strongly suggest that organisms that have achieved such symbiotic relationships have been associated during their evolutionary development and have become thereby not only interdependent but exquisitely adapted to each other.

Lichens illustrate the immense value of symbiosis in the plant kingdom. These symbiotic organisms exist in a great number of varieties – on the surface of rocks, on tree trunks, even in the Arctic and Antarctic wastes and other places that appear completely unsuitable for the maintenance of life. Lichens owe their ability to survive and to proliferate under such desolate conditions to their symbiotic nature. They are made up of two different microbial species, an alga and a fungus, which are closely interwoven and interdependent. The alga and the fungus that constitute a lichen complement each other in their chemical and physiological attributes. As a result, the lichen can derive nutriment from situations where neither the alga nor the fungus could have subsisted alone. Furthermore, it can resist noxious conditions, such as heat, cold or drought, that would be fatal to either partner alone. Even more interestingly, the association results in the production of new structures characteristic of a lichen, structures that often display vivid colours and a great morphological beauty that neither the alga nor the fungus produces when growing alone.

Symbiosis is evident also in the intestinal tract of animals, including man. The intestine normally harbours immense numbers of various kinds of bacteria. It was long believed that these intestinal microorganisms were accidental intruders, either totally insignificant or potentially dangerous. Recent experiments have shown, however, that certain types of bacteria, always present in the gastrointestinal tract of healthy animals or persons, do in fact play a highly beneficial role. They are essential for the full development of their host; they contribute to his nutrition; and they increase his resistance to various stresses, including disease. Reciprocally, the gastrointestinal tract of the host provides conditions suitable for the multiplication of the beneficial bacteria. In other words, microbe and man (in this instance) exist in a symbiotic relationship.

In the preceding paragraphs, we have selected the two extreme ends of the Great Chain of Being, microbe and man, to illustrate the biological interest of symbiotic relationships. It is worth emphasizing, however, that the phenomenon of interspecies dependence is not a biological rarity, but is encountered throughout nature and involves all kinds of organisms. The widespread occurrence of symbiotic association is not a mere academic curiosity; it has enormous practical importance because it accounts for the profound and often disastrous consequences that follow any upset in the balance of nature.

Rachel Carson's book *Silent Spring* publicized the fact that thoughtless use of pesticides can bring about the death of birds (which feed on poisoned insects) and can in more general ways upset the balance of nature. The larger significance of her warning is that any measure that grossly alters natural conditions is likely also to have indirect unfavourable effects because all components of nature are interrelated and interdependent. While the phrase 'chain of being' remains useful for describing the hierarchical order of living forms, it fails to convey the complexity of their ecological relationships. From the functional point of view, the different living forms are organized not as a chain but as a highly integrated web, only as strong as the weakest of its constituent threads.

The interdependence of living forms and their complex relation to the physical environment constitute critical factors in the development of conservation policies. Man is dependent not only on other human beings and on the physical world but also on the other creatures – animals, plants and microbes – that have evolved together with him. Man will ultimately destroy himself if he thoughtlessly eliminates the organisms that constitute essential links in the complex and delicate web of life of which he is a part.

Socialization and Learned Behaviour Among Animals

Communities consisting of different animal species living together under natural conditions have evolved regulatory mechanisms of a social nature that maintain order and balance among them. These mechanisms are the result of various compensatory feedback processes that became established in the course of evolutionary development and are therefore largely automatic and unconscious.

The population of any given animal species also exhibits social regulatory mechanisms. The hierarchical order that develops among the various members of the species is the expression of automatic mechanisms supplemented by learned behaviour patterns. The more one studies animal behaviour, the more apparent it becomes that many essential activities depend upon learning while young. Learned behaviour is of greater importance in the socialization of higher animal species, especially of the primates. It reaches its greatest significance in the social development of man.

The simultaneous presence of several members of a given animal species in one area does not suffice to define a society. A true social order implies communication among the individual members; the integration of their activities; and the subordination of their separate interests to those of the group. Fulfilment of these criteria always requires the operation of innate forces governing the responses of one animal to the others. In most species this instinctive endowment is supplemented by a learned behaviour transferred from one animal to the other and from one generation to the next.

In many respects, the beehive presents one of the most highly organized and successful types of social structure. Everything that happens in the hive serves its community as a whole, and its management depends upon an elaborate system of communication among individual honeybees. For this reason, many attempts have been made to derive from the life of the bees lessons applicable to human life.

Although the beehive constitutes a remarkable biological

achievement, profound differences in its familial pattern seriously limit its relevance to human societal organization. For one thing, a community of honeybees is made up not of an association of families but of one single huge family whose population may reach 80,000 individuals. The contrast to human societies, which consist of multiple familial units with great genetic diversity, is obvious. Furthermore, the beehive is governed by inborn urges that manifest themselves in the form of rigidly fixed behaviour patterns, whereas the dominant characteristic of human societies is that they are forever changing their environment, their ways of life, and ultimately their very organization. Another peculiarity of honeybees, as well as of other social insects such as termites, is that they represent highly specialized and perhaps terminal types of evolution. It is, therefore, of greater human interest to study the social patterns of mammalian species that are more closely related to man.

One can find in various animal species models for most, if not all, social situations encountered in human life. The reason these analogies can exist is that the emergence of new characteristics during evolution does not necessarily entail the complete disappearance of more ancient ones. The genetic endowment is modified during evolutionary development but is never entirely lost. In man, for example, the most sophisticated expressions of reflective consciousness coexist with the irrational impulses and the elemental forms of conditioning that dominate the life of more primitive creatures. All aspects of human life, individual and social, exhibit some of the characteristics found not only in our primate relatives but also in our more remote evolutionary ancestors. The recent events associated with the two world wars have made it painfully obvious that, whenever the environmental conditions are somewhat analogous to those of the distant past, primitive urges and reaction patterns can rapidly break through the thin layer of civil behaviour developed by man under peacetime conditions.

The use of language is the one characteristic most commonly regarded as differentiating man from animals. It is true that animals are not, as far as we can judge, able to engage in abstract symbolism and therefore have not the equivalent of human language. Without doubt, however, they can communicate very effectively through, for example, the use of sounds, scents or gestures. The 'dance' language of the bees transmits precise information to other bees concerning the direction and distance of a food source. But such language is innate, not learned; moreover, there is no evidence that it represents a conscious intention to communicate. The same limitations apparently apply also to birdcall notes. Small birds take cover from a hawk or other predators when they hear the alarm call uttered by one of their own species. Thus they show that they have 'understood' the message, but the call and the response to it seem to be purely instinctive. No conscious assessment on the part of the bird is apparently involved. Parrots can learn to articulate sounds and imitate the human voice, but there is no evidence whatever that they can use any language syntactically.

As one ascends the evolutionary scale, animal communications begin to resemble human communications. In many situations higher mammals behave as if they were trying to express true purposive behaviour when they utter certain sounds or display certain gestures. In *The Expression of the Emotions in Man and Animals*, Charles Darwin described an impressive series of communication behaviour patterns revealing similarities between animals and men. Uncovering the canine tooth communicates 'hostility', as does spitting and the ejection of the tongue; erection of hair and dilation of pupils signal 'fear'; raising the body to an erect position can symbolize the 'sense of pride'. Modern research has greatly extended Darwin's pioneering observations and brought to light many subtle gestures and attitudes of communication in animals, especially among primates.

Whether modes of communication among animals bear any real relation to human language and provide clues to its origin is still undecided at present. Common sense tells us that no animal has developed or can learn to use a language as propositional, as syntactic, and as clearly expressive of complex intentions as the language of man. As logical as this view seems, it is nevertheless an assumption so far not testable, and may be just an expression of our human conceit. There is suggestive evidence, furthermore, that most, if not all, the features of human languages can be found separately, in a more or less primitive form, in one or another of the animal species.

Instinct unquestionably controls most means of communication used by animals. On the other hand, even among birds, and more so among mammals, the repertoire of sounds they utter or of signs and gestures they make, and to which they respond, can be markedly increased by conditioning or by trial and error – in other words, by learning. Furthermore, higher animals can learn improved communicating skills that they can use in their familial and social behaviour. Little doubt exists, for example, that when wild female animals have learned to fear man from unpleasant experience, they develop new patterns of protective behaviour and teach their young to recognize special warning signals associated with the approach of human beings.

It must be acknowledged at this point that, surprising as it may seem, the scientific definition of the word 'learning' presents great conceptual difficulties to professional psychologists. The word is used here somewhat loosely, as in general conversation, to denote any change in adaptive behaviour resulting from experience. In this broad sense, learned behaviour occurs throughout the animal kingdom; moreover, it can take forms of increasing complexity, ranging from that exhibited by very primitive organisms without a nervous system to that found in higher apes and, of course, in man.

At one end of the spectrum, the learning process can be illustrated by an experiment carried out with a protozoan. One of these primitive unicellular creatures was exposed to an acid concentration so weak as not to affect its behaviour; then the acid concentration was raised to an injurious level. After the experiment had been repeated several times, the protozoan learned and remembered from prior experience that contact with a solution not injurious in itself foretold of exposure to a stronger, dangerous acid concentration. The experienced protozoan took advantage of this awareness to escape in advance of the approach of danger. The faculty for learning is so highly developed even among simple organisms that it makes them respond to the symbols of danger as vigorously as to the stimulus itself.

Learned patterns of behaviour become increasingly important as one ascends the ladder of life. Wild animals display little fear of travellers in areas where they have little contact with man or where he is not allowed to harm them, for example, in unexplored regions, in national parks, or in game preserves. However, they avoid man when their collective experience has taught them to consider him a potential enemy. Animal behaviour is conditioned by social memory.

The most elaborate forms of learned behaviour have been observed, as might be expected, among the higher primates. A chimpanzee, for example, can learn to pile up boxes and climb on them – or to use a stick – to obtain bananas placed at a height otherwise beyond its reach. Moreover, other apes that have observed such complex behaviour rapidly learn to duplicate it by imitation.

Higher animals often behave as if they were deliberately aiming at some immediate end that they have thought out. In many cases, indeed, their activities suggest that they engage in abstract ideation; they behave as if they had the faculty to create images in the absence of any corresponding external stimulus. The chimpanzee mentioned above could 'see' in advance the possibility of reaching the banana with a stick. This kind of insight learning is probably based on trial-and-error manipulation of ideas. It involves the solution of problems through an adaptive reorganization of experience and may be closely related to conscious understanding in man.

Under natural conditions, many mechanisms are available to the young animal for acquiring new kinds of information and new skills to supplement those provided by instinct. For example, all higher animals exhibit during their early lives a great propensity to explore their environments as well as to engage in play and even in intricate games. The extent of the curiosity to explore and the complexity of play seem to have a direct relation to the degree of mental development of the animal species. It is obvious that in young animals, as in human infants, all forms of exploration and of play facilitate acquaintance with the external world, accelerate the development of physical and mental skills, and probably extend the perceptual horizon.

The most essential attitudes and skills of every animal species are acquired during the very early stages of life. The duckling thus becomes attached by 'imprinting' to the first object it perceives after emerging from the egg. This object may be a stick, a man, or another duck; but in nature the first thing that the duckling perceives, fortunately, is the mother duck. This phenomenon of imprinting is extremely pronounced in birds and can be regarded almost as a caricature of the profound effects exerted by early influences on the subsequent behaviour of animals and men. Since the mother is normally the newborn's first contact, she accounts for most of the influences that condition early development. Students of animal behaviour have made fascinating observations on the elaborate techniques used by female animals to teach their young such essential skills as how to fly, swim, find food, learn danger signals and run for shelter.

Many unpredictable things happen to animals, among them contact with man, hunters in particular, or change in the kind of available food. Survival therefore often depends on their ability to learn new kinds of behaviour. Transmission of acquired skills to the young is generally more important among mammals than among birds, whose lives are quite stereotyped. Furthermore, some mammals are born without elementary skills; infant fur seals cannot swim, and the pet lioness Elsa[1] could not hunt. In most mammals such skills are learned from the parents. Learned behaviour, transmitted from the parents

1. Joy Adamson, *Born Free*, Collins, 1962.

to the young, thus constitutes the rudiments of culture in the animal kingdom.

Almost as important as the role of the mother in behavioural and even physiological development is association with other young animals. Young mammals raised in isolation, and thus deprived of the chance to play with their peers, later exhibit profoundly abnormal behaviour when they meet others of their species. For example, primates kept isolated for several weeks after birth show obvious signs of neurosis and fail to engage in sexual activity when they are caged with sexually mature animals of the opposite sex. If, perchance, a female that has been isolated during childhood becomes pregnant, either she neglects her firstborn or mistreats it. Even so, she can learn from experience.

The influences that condition physiological and behavioural development naturally differ in important details from species to species. In all cases, nonetheless, the individual members of animal societies living under natural conditions eventually become integrated by a multiplicity of behaviour patterns. Some of these patterns are truly instinctive; they are built up in the hereditary endowment. Others, as we have seen, are acquired early in life and transmitted by learning from one generation to the next. Still others are acquired later in life as a result of the interplay between adult animals. We shall now consider two types of social behaviour – territoriality and dominance – that greatly contribute to the socialization of the group and increase its adaptation to its environment.

Territoriality and Dominance

Animal populations living in a given area develop complex social structures for the control of territory and hierarchical organization. The size of the group, the extent of its territory, and the type of hierarchical organization are characteristic for each species, as are the means by which the animals communicate with each other and thus develop their social structure. The croaking of frogs, the song of birds, the howling of monkeys, and even the language of dolphins certainly play a role in establishing territorial claims and social status. Many other physiological characteristics and behavioural traits have a definite social meaning. For instance, the deposition of secretions, excretions or other odorous substances at selected spots serves to mark territorial boundaries. Certain physical attributes or forms of display also contribute to the establishment of dominance within a given territory and social group.

Irrespective of the nature of its determinants, social organization has several important beneficial effects. It generates mechanisms that regulate population size more or less automatically; it limits the severity of conflicts within the group; and in many cases it prevents destructive combat except in unusual or unnatural situations.

Whenever the population density of a group increases beyond a safe limit, many of the low-ranking animals in the social hierarchy are removed from the reproductive pool. Some are chased out and compelled to emigrate; others are tolerated on the fringes of the group but not allowed to engage in heterosexual activity, becoming, as it were, social castrates.

That only the most vigorous and otherwise most able males have access to the females probably has some eugenic value; it tends to favour reproduction of genes responsible for physical and behavioural vigour. Notwithstanding, the greatest importance of forced emigration and of social castration is to limit the number of males available for mating and thus to prevent excessive population growth. The population-limiting effect of this social mechanism supplements that exerted by food shortages and by other selective biological processes. The remarkable outcome of these automatic mechanisms is that, in the case of many animal species, animal populations in the wild remain on the average much more stable than would be expected from the maximum reproductive potential. Automatic regulatory mechanisms of population size, involving both biological and social factors, have been found to operate also among animal populations maintained in laboratory environments.

Since the patterns of behaviour based on territoriality and social hierarchy have emerged in the course of evolutionary development it can be taken for granted that they possess some adaptive value, if not for each individual member at least for the group as a whole. Studies of animal behaviour have revealed that fighting and social tensions subside once the hierarchical order is established and accepted, and that competition for food and for mates is abated. The group thus enjoys a social stability beneficial not only to its dominant members but also to the subordinate animals. Admittedly, the latter must yield their places to dominant animals in the feeding areas and consequently do not grow as rapidly as they otherwise would. On the other hand, these behaviour patterns, along with the restrictions imposed by territoriality, limit the numbers of animals breeding in a given area and thereby maintain an equilibrium between the population and its food resources. Such biological checks on food consumption are consonant with the belief of conservationists that exploitation of natural resources should remain somewhat below maximum utilization.

The population regulatory mechanisms mentioned above operate effectively because many members of the group are deprived of a chance to reproduce and others are sacrificed altogether. At first sight, therefore, it seems paradoxical to assert that the behavioural patterns involved in territoriality and dominance have adaptive value. By defining Darwinian fitness with reference to the population as a whole rather than to the individual organism, we can explain the paradox. In contrast, civilized human societies, and probably most primitive human societies as well, tend to regard the individual person as the significant biological unit. This difference sharply separates mankind from the rest of the living world and explains why many social mechanisms effective among animals are ethically unacceptable in human societies. For this reason, the automatic regulatory processes that control numbers of animals in nature are of limited importance in controlling the human population.

The pecking order among chickens and other birds, as well as other forms of hierarchical arrangement in animal societies, depends upon the ability of some animals to establish dominance over subordinate members of the group. For a long time it was thought that dominance was achieved through fierce combat, in particular when males were in conflict for the available females during the rut season. Savage fights between stags, walrus bulls or male seals have long been part of wildlife lore. However, destructive combat rarely occurs under natural conditions; it is rare also among laboratory animals if the colony is left undisturbed once it has become stabilized. When males fight, the combat rarely is to the death. The stronger combatant intimidates and threatens, the weaker turns aside and retreats. The victor lets the vanquished flee unmolested.

The losing animal in a struggle saves itself from destruction by an act of submission, an act usually recognized and accepted by the winner. In some cases, for instance, the loser presents to its rival a vulnerable part of its body such as the top of the head or the fleshy part of the neck. The central nervous system of the winner recognizes the 'meaning' of the presentation, and the instinct to kill is inhibited. Typical of this natural pattern is the behaviour of two wolves in combat. As soon as one of the animals realizes it cannot win, it offers its vulnerable throat to the stronger wolf; instead of taking advantage of the opportunity, the victor relents, even though an instant earlier it had appeared frantic to reach the now proffered jugular vein. Many fish that 'fight' do not actually strike each other; they merely beat their tails in a way that creates shock waves of water against the sensitive lateral line of the other. To the observer this performance resembles more closely a complex ritual than a real fight.

The view that destructive combat is rare among wild animals is so much at variance with the 'Nature, red in tooth and claw' legend that it may be useful to quote here a statement by Professor Niko Tinbergen, a well-known student of ethology, or animal behaviour: 'It is a very striking and important fact that "fighting" in animals usually consists of threatening or bluff. Considering the fact that sexual fighting takes such an enormous amount of the time (in the breeding season) of so many species, it is certainly astonishing that real fighting, in the sense of a physical struggle, is so seldom observed.'[2]

In some respects, fighting among animals under natural conditions thus presents some analogy to German student duels; some wounds are permissible, but most battles constitute in reality bluffing contests and a confrontation of wits. As far as is known, only one type of creature in addition to man engages in systematic destructive war against other groups of the same species. At times when food is scarce among harvester ants, colonies of these ants are prone to raid those other colonies of the same species that have stored away seeds; they kill the owners and carry away the crop. It need not be emphasized that among men also war has often been waged for a food supply.

An extensive symposium on the symbolic nature of fighting between animals of the same species was recently held in London under the title 'The Ritualization of Behaviour'. This symposium noted that animals repeatedly tend to ritualize their aggression by such conduct as rearing up, roaring, showing their teeth, or erecting their ruffs, hackles, or neck hair. Since ritualization of behaviour is widespread also among higher apes, it is surprising that man differs from them, as well as from most other animals, in having practised warfare extensively with the intent to kill. History and contemporary events unfortunately leave no doubt that man is a killer, but the reason for this propensity is not readily found in evolutionary development.[3] A few facts having a possible relevance to this problem seem worth mentioning here because

2. *Biology, Psychology, and Belief*, Cambridge University Press, 1961.

3. For some interesting and provocative notions of man's legacy of aggression, see Robert Ardrey, *The Territorial Imperative*, Atheneum, New York, 1966, and Konrad Lorenz, *On Aggression*, Harcourt, Brace & World, New York, English trans. 1966.

they may point to the nature of the social mechanisms that have made man the only creature among the higher animals who will systematically engage in destructive internecine warfare.

Although war is extremely rare among animals living in the wild, naturally one finds a few exceptions to the rule of 'bluff rather than fight'. For example, when an animal enters the home ground of another member of the same species, the latter attacks at once, apparently with the intent to kill the intruder. Such hostile attitudes apply chiefly or only to animals of the same species; other animals with slightly different habits or nutritional needs are usually not considered as competitors, and their presence is tolerated. Thus the concept of the stranger seems to have had its origins in the fear of losing one's place in the sun to potential competitors for the available food and mates. The concept of foreigners in human life – along with the undertones of mistrust and fear associated with the word in all languages – may well have its biological origin in the hostile reaction of animals to strangers of their own kind moving into their own territory.

Comparative observations of primates living undisturbed in their natural habitats or in zoos have thrown further light on the possible social mechanisms through which man became a killer. When primates live under natural conditions, territory is held in common by each band and is respected by the neighbour bands. Each individual animal within the band has right of access to the common territory. Order is maintained by a hierarchy of ranks evolved as each generation grows up. This hierarchy is subject to rearrangement in accordance with the strength of the leaders and with their performance in guiding and protecting the rest of the band. The leader of a primate society settles quarrels within the band before they become violent and even gives evidence of a realistic respect for the rights of neighbouring bands. Furthermore, the bonds of comradeship holding the wild society together are far more prominent in day-to-day life than are occasional episodes of pulling rank.

Regulatory mechanisms of peaceful interplay within the

band break down when animals find themselves in environments unlike those in which they have evolved. In zoos, for example, especially in old, poorly designed ones, where animals are crowded, they have little opportunity for exploring and for the individualistic enterprise they normally exercise in the wild. In such an environment the selection of the group leader is no longer dependent on his having the ability for real leadership, as it is in the wild. As no food shortage exists in the zoo, an ape community there may become comparable to an urban human society, crowded and without tradition, yet enjoying material abundance.

Whenever primates are under crowded conditions, rank becomes established through fighting, and the wrong animals are likely to come to the top. They do not have to meet the test of useful performance in solving the problems of the band, and they commonly try to maintain their authority by threats or actual acts of violence. Quarrels between individual animals may become endemic, and now and then the whole society collapses. Females and young may be indiscriminately slaughtered in such outbreaks of violence. In brief, primates under crowded conditions, as they sometimes are in zoos, commonly treat their fellow inmates with extreme cruelty, but animals of the same species give no evidence of vicious behaviour when they live in their natural environment

The observations made on primates probably have some bearing on the human condition. When man emerged from his animal background, he created for himself an environment and ways of life in which the social restraints achieved during his evolutionary development were no longer effective or suitable. Biological adaptation had not prepared him for the competitive attitudes that characterized his new social relations. He became a killer of his own species when he began to create new competitive social structures without developing social restraints to substitute for the biological wisdom of animal life evolved under natural conditions. Even today, violence and internecine conflicts are most common in highly competitive societies, particularly during periods of rapid change. Man has not yet learned to live in the zoo he has created for himself.

One of the most urgent needs of human life is to invent new ways of ritualizing social conflicts. Fortunately, this may not be as impossible as it appears at first sight. After all, the jousts between medieval knights, and some of the later traditions of military behaviour, were comparable to the sham fights so common among animal populations in the wild; no one doubts that these battles of bravado averted countless wider conflicts. Can contemporary society develop effective techniques for the ritualization of conflicts? Is it too naïve to assume that global games (like the Olympics) and political confrontations can substitute for war? Competition in education and technology – or even in social welfare – can perhaps serve to evoke national potentialities that have often found their greatest expression in war's demanding and often stirring call to heroism. The race to the moon, and other forms of space exploration, may be modern expressions of what William James called the moral equivalent for war. If these sublimations of aggression can substitute for war, is any expenditure too great?

Nature, Nurture and the Biological Past

Whether they be plants or animals, microbial cells or human beings, all living organisms develop and function under the control of the genes they inherit. In consequence, all the traits that determine the physical and mental personality of each particular organism, and that differentiate it from all others, are unquestionably under the control of the instructions inscribed in the genetic code. While size and shape, physiological functions, and behavioural patterns are all conditioned by heredity, these attributes are also obviously influenced by diet, climate, social milieu, and countless other factors of the environment. Creatures identical in genetic constitution, such as identical twins, nevertheless differ markedly if they are reared under dissimilar conditions.

The genetic and environmental points of view thus provide two distinct approaches to the study of living processes. Indeed, at first sight they appear to yield biological philosophies that are so different as to be incompatible. In reality, both are correct and both necessary for an understanding of life.

Recent findings point to a possible cellular mechanism to explain the obvious but puzzling fact that the characteristics of an organism are determined both by its genetic constitution and by the forces of its environment. In brief, it has been found that only a small percentage of the genes are in an active state in any particular organism at any given time. Environmental forces can set in motion within the organism certain physiologcal processes that determine which parts of the genetic code are activated. The ancient controversy that had for so long put nature and nurture in opposition arose from incomplete knowledge of the intimate mechanisms of life. Modern genetic theory has confirmed the commonsense view that, while the potential expressions of organisms are determined by their hereditary endowment, the environment regulates the manner and extent to which these potentialities are expressed during life.

In broad outline, two different kinds of influences thus play a role in determining the 'nature' of the organism. On the one hand, each organism acquires the accumulated effects of the evolutionary past as embodied in the genes. On the other hand, each organism acquires, through mechanisms that do not alter its genetic code, characteristics determined by stimuli that affect it during its own lifetime. Thus, the effects of the experential past exist side by side with those of the evolutionary past. Whether they modify the responses of the body (as in allergic sensitization) or of the psyche (as in emotional reactions), most forms of experiential conditioning are extremely lasting. The child who has been sensitized to poison ivy is likely to remain sensitive thereafter; similarly, the memories of early youth may remain influential and even vivid until old age. Skills and concepts acquired during childhood are rarely completely lost. Some of the imprints of the experiential past do indeed persist throughout the whole life-span.

Prenatal and early postnatal influences are particularly important because they have such a profound and lasting effect on the physical and mental characteristics of the child and adult. For example, nutritional and emotional deprivations suffered by newborn animals during the formative period almost inevitably result in developmental and behavioural defects; many of these can never be completely erased. Stresses experienced by the mother during the early phases of gestation can also cause irreversible abnormalities in the young. Public attention has been attracted to this problem by the thalidomide tragedy. In the more complete picture, nutritional deficiencies and emotional disturbances, as well as exposure to toxic agents, including many kinds of drugs, can indirectly influence the foetus through effects on the mother. There is then a rudiment of truth in the old wives' tales that the pregnant woman's emotions and experiences during gestation can have unfavourable effects on the child.

Living organisms thus differ from inanimate matter by the extent to which their development and responses are determined by their total history. In this regard, the biological persistence of the past gives a profound meaning to the phrase inscribed on the shield of the hero in Tennyson's poem 'Ulysses' – 'I am a part of all that I have met.' Life is historical. Furthermore, each being creates more history as it moves in its environment, responds to it, and is thereby irreversibly altered.

The view of biology as history might be construed as an intellectual distortion resulting from overemphasis on human problems. In reality, the historical aspects of life are just as important for simple organisms as they are for the higher ones and for man. The effects of the organism's biological history on the responses that it makes to environmental stimuli do not constitute fashionable subjects of investigation, probably because they cannot as yet be analysed by physico-chemical methods. Popular or not, such studies are of immense interest because manifestations of behaviour at primitive levels of organization present analogies to those encountered in human life. The following observations made on sea urchins bear out the pertinence of such analogies.

Although a sea urchin tends to remain in dark places, a sudden darker shadow falling on its body stimulates it to point its spines toward the object casting the shadow. The reaction is elicited by the shadow, but it refers to something symbolized by the shadow, the imminence of a possible predator. The sea urchin's response to a shadow is evidence that, even in the case of relatively primitive animals, behaviour is conditioned by the ancient experiences of the species. This response to shadows constitutes a symbol of all the indelible imprints that the past has left on the sea urchin.

Similar symbolic reactions reach a complex development in higher animals, In man, most responses to things seen, heard, or felt are essentially reactions to symbolic stimuli.

Mutations constantly occur in all living organisms, and continuous environmental changes provide endless opportunities for the selection of new types arising from the reshuffling of the hereditary endowment. Mutations are accidental, chance events, but selection constitutes a kind of antichance force. It acts as a sieve that retains only those attributes best suited to the prevailing environmental conditions. To this extent, evolution is a creative process since it provides an order and a pattern for the preservation, accumulation and organization of the best preadapted mutants.

Evolutionary doctrine provides at present the only available explanation based on natural laws for the progressive emergence of new forms of life, but the history of science makes it very probable that orthodox Darwinism will eventually reveal internal contradictions, as have all scientific theories in the past. One can take it for granted that the future will reveal many biological facts outside evolutionary concepts as we know them today, requiring a more sophisticated reformulation of these concepts.

Even in its present crude form, however, the theory of evolution provides a rational explanation for the existence of a progressive order of complexity, beginning with the lowest animals and extending to man. The order that the ancients perceived and symbolized by the images of the 'ladder of life' or the Great Chain of Being is in truth an expression of natural forces.

Whatever the precise mechanisms through which it operates, evolutionary development seems to have been accompanied by a gradual integration of the different sensory systems. In all animals each sensory organ has its own centre of coordination. This is true of even lower animals, such as flatworms, sea anemones, or starfishes. In these forms the central nervous system is poorly developed. As a result, lower animals give the impression of being hardly integrated at all. The higher the animal on the evolutionary scale, the more complex its central nervous system and the more complete its integration.

The integrative process reaches its culmination in adult man. Like the young of all higher animals, the human infant at birth lacks the ability to recognize objects and fails to search for them after they disappear from view; these aptitudes are acquired. The mind as a unifying and integrating entity seems to be a late product of individual as well as of evolutionary development.

For reasons that are far from clear, the ability to coordinate sense impressions is associated with a number of other attributes. Many of the higher animals exhibit something like a fundamental drive to perceive. They tend to codify all the impressions they secure through their visual, auditory or other senses into a total picture of the external world. This tendency seems to be related to some kind of curiosity organized around the activities of the sense organs.

As evolutionary development brings about an increasing elaboration of the nervous system and of its associated sense organs, it also renders animals increasingly independent of environmental forces and progressively more capable of altering the environment to their own ends. Whether or not these evolutionary changes – revolutionary in the long run – constitute real progress is a question beyond the scope of biological knowledge alone. What is certain is that independence from environmental factors and the ability to manipulate these factors are attributes that have reached their highest level in man. In this respect, at least, man unquestionably occupies the highest position on the ladder of life on earth. Indeed, the life of man, although not his body, differs so much from that of other animals that he must in practice be considered apart from them. As we shall see, one of the great unsolved problems of biology is to explain why man is so profoundly different from other organisms even though he is so obviously linked to them in the Great Chain of Being.

2 Man's Nature

Man's Dual Nature

Man, as a member of the animal kingdom, is by evolutionary descent directly linked to other living things and indirectly related to inanimate matter. In the words of Paul the Apostle, 'The first man is of the earth, earthy.' But human life as we know it today is so far removed from its earthy and animal origins that it poses problems not found in the rest of creation. While man is an animal, obviously he is an extraordinary animal whose life has unique characteristics. In the present chapter we shall have to keep in mind constantly these two contrasting aspects of man's nature, his animal attributes, and the humanness of his life.

Recognizing man when we encounter him, either in ancient documents or in remote places, presents no problem. None of our present knowledge, however, enables us to identify adequately the biological characteristics that account for his uniqueness. He does not possess any noteworthy genetic or developmental singularity not already foreshadowed in lower forms. The ability to walk erect, the liberation of the forelimbs for manipulation, the crossing over of the optic tracts and binocular vision, the enlargement of the cerebral cortex, and the prolongation of childhood are all important biological characteristics of man. But these characteristics are not biological innovations of the human species; they are merely exaggerations of tendencies seen in all apes.

Toolmaking, social organization, communication with other members of the group, acquisition and transmission of learned behaviour – are skills without which man could not survive but which also exist to some degree in various lower animal species. Even such complex mental attributes as ideation (the ability to symbolize) and altruism appear in primitive form among higher animals. A man can reach full development only through association with other men, but the need for affective communication and for affiliation also exists as an instinct among higher animals and is almost as primary as other biological drives.

In brief, man is characterized less by his biological and social endowments than by what he has created from them. He differs from the rest of the animal kingdom chiefly through his collective achievements over several thousands of generations. In this light, the statement, by the Spanish philosopher Ortega y Gasset, that 'Man ... has no nature, what he has is ... history' finds much justification; but this epigram does nothing more, unfortunately, than restate the problem. We would like to know what peculiarities of man's nature have enabled him to have a history.

Human life is the product of the social and cultural forces that have made history. In addition, the history of each person encompasses his evolutionary past and his private biological experiences. Moreover, environmental forces affecting the biological characteristics of its members profoundly influence the history of each social group. From one point of view, man appears as an extremely complex assembly of organic materials whose fundamental composition and properties are similar to those found in all other livings things and even in non-living matter. For this reason, the human body can be studied as a machine, the structures and mechanisms of which obey the laws of physics and chemistry. From another point of view, man is seen as a complex organism, exhibiting unique responses to his environment not readily accounted for by the phenomena observed in inanimate matter or in the rest of the living world. Man's responses are determined less by the direct effects of external stimuli on his body fabric than by the symbolic interpretation attached by each individual person to these stimuli. The models and symbols through which the human mind operates are derived from the external world, but they eventually acquire a life of their own largely independent of their factual origin.

Thus man's nature comprises two profoundly different but complementary aspects. Most attributes of the body machine are common to all members of the species *Homo sapiens* and almost identical with those of higher apes; they can be successfully studied by the orthodox methods of the natural sciences. At the same time, each person has peculiarities deriving from his own experiences and activities, special traits that make him different from all other persons. These attributes are not readily amenable to scientific analysis because science deals ineffectively with unique events. General scientific laws can be formulated for the species *Homo sapiens*, but they are never sufficient to account for the uniqueness of individual human beings and of their achievements.

As we shall emphasize repeatedly, it is all but impossible to define or describe the biological characteristics that differentiate *Homo sapiens* from other animals, and each person from all other persons. Both individual and collective differences are extremely subtle, and involve complex patterns rather than unit structures or functions. Furthermore, an enumeration of them cannot give a complete picture of reality. Mankind progressively disappears in the analytical process and can be apprehended only as a whole. This is as true of the individual as of the human race.

Scientists have made definite progress towards identifying the environmental forces that in the past progressively differentiated mankind from the animal kingdom and today contribute to the uniqueness of each individual human being. To illustrate the power of these forces, we shall consider in the following pages how man's nature reflects the moulding influence of the physical and social environment. Anthropological evidence makes it probable that the precursors of *Homo sapiens*, and their ways of life, developed simultaneously during geological times through a long and complex series of feedback processes. In a somewhat analogous manner, each human being now acquires a large part of his personality through his responses to the total environment, especially during the early formative years of his life. Man's nature cannot be described fully in terms of static, fixed characteristics; it is best understood as an expression of responses to the influences experienced during the evolutionary and experiential past.

When applied to living systems, the word evolution can designate phenomena as different as the physical and mental development of individual persons; the Darwinian transformation of biological species; and the progressive alterations of social and economic structures. In all these cases, evolution refers to the long-range moulding of the biological or social system by environmental forces, usually as a result of learning by experience. This process of change can occur only through a variety of mechanisms having little in common.

Even when the problem is considered from a purely biological point of view, the variations exhibited by living organisms fall into two distinct categories: genetic mutations, which affect the very substance of the hereditary material located in the chromosomes; phenotypic modifications, which do not alter the genetic constitution but arise from responses of the whole organism to environmental factors. According to the classical formulation of the neo-Darwinian theory, genetic mutations and their selection by the environment account for progressive changes undergone by biological species and for the emergence of new species; phenotypic modifications affect only the individual organism. It is becoming apparent, however, that the interplay between organism and environment is far more subtle than indicated by this formulation. As pointed out by the geneticist C. H. Waddington 'modes of behavior ... combine with external circumstances to determine the nature of the effective environment'.

It is a truism that a given environment can act as a selective agent and thus govern evolutionary changes only if the animal elects to stay and function in it long enough to reproduce. In general, an animal elects a given environment because it can respond to it by successful phenotypic adaptations. This oversimplified statement of an immensely complex problem will suffice to suggest that the evolutionary system embraces a dual concept: it comprises not only the mutations and selective pressures of classical neo-Darwinism but also the processes by which animals, men in particular, choose and modify one particular habitat out of all the environmental possibilities open to them.

This modern view of biological evolution appears in some respects to be based on the discredited Lamarckian hypothesis that any sustained form of activity will eventually bring about a corresponding physical or mental change, transmissible from parent to offspring. Without doubt this interpretation is erroneous, and biological evolution is always mediated through genetic and selective agencies. The point to be emphasized here is that all evolutionary phenomena involve feedback processes between the organism, its environment, and its ways of life. It will be helpful to illustrate this concept with two examples taken from the nonhuman world.

The shape of certain flowers is exquisitely adapted to the insects that feed on them and thereby act as pollinators for them. This high degree of adaptive fitness between flower and pollinator certainly required long periods of evolutionary development during which the plant responded to the stimulus of the feeding organs of the insect. For example, the clover flower 'appears' to have developed its anatomical characteristics by 'responding' to the bumblebee; similarly, the flower of the trumpet vine appears to have evolved in response to the hummingbird. The study of plant and animal fossils, however, suggests that the mutual adaptations between flowers and insects or birds have origins even more distant and more subtle. The modern view is that flowers, and their insect or bird visitors, have evolved simultaneously from primitive forms. In the early stages of their development they had become loosely associated long before they had reached their present state of evolutionary development. Insects and birds, in the very process of developing their own behavioural patterns, nutritional habits and feeding organs, would thus have determined the characteristics of the flowers on which they feed and which they pollinate. Mutual adaptations would have developed through a series of feedbacks between plants and pollinators, seesaw fashion.

The social behaviour of chimpanzees and gorillas provides further evidence for the operation of cybernetic mechanisms in evolutionary development. In their undisturbed forest habitats, adult chimpanzees do not become organized in families, harems, or other types of stable social structures. Individual chimpanzees move rapidly over large areas, often in fairly numerous bands but without leaders and without permanent associations. In contrast, gorillas live in small permanent groups; the members of each group keep in contact with each other all the time and are led usually by a big silver-backed male. The anthropologist Vernon Reynolds, who observed chimpanzees and gorillas in the African forest, believes that the differences in social organization between these two species can be traced to their food habits. In his words, the chimpanzees are 'happiest when they gorge themselves on fruits for hours at a time, high in the tree tops'. Since they subsist chiefly on large fruits, they must scatter over large areas in order to find enough to eat; hence their fluid and dispersed social organization. Unlike chimpanzees, gorillas are herbivorous rather than frugivorous; pithy stems, leaves, roots and bark are their main sources of food, fruits providing no more than a supplement. Constantly surrounded by abundant food in their lush tropical environment, they can feed as they go without moving far and can maintain a stable social organization. Eventually, the behaviour patterns and determinants of social organization characteristic of the chimpanzees and the gorillas became embodied in the respective genetic codes of these two species.

Lamarck believed that the organism's behaviour determines to a large extent the environmental situation in which it develops and to which its offspring become adapted. The theory that nutritional habits and tastes have been influential in determining the social organization of chimpanzees and gorillas therefore has Lamarckian overtones. As shown by Wadding-

ton, this semi-Lamarckian interpretation of population genetics is but a cybernetic extension of the neo-Darwinian doctrine that evolutionary changes occur through the agency of
mutations and selection. This cybernetic concept appears compatible with many facts of human evolution. As we shall now
see, it is probable that the environments into which man's
precursors moved during the Paleolithic period conditioned
the activities in which they engaged, and this in turn eventually
determined the genetic endowment that now characterizes
mankind.

Man's Evolutionary Past

Even the most superficial observer perceives that man is related to other animals, especially to the higher apes, but
scholars differ concerning the precise nature of this relationship. Most biologists are naturally impressed by the continuity
so evident throughout the living world and focus their attention on those aspects of man that reveal him the product of
an unbroken evolutionary trend. They believe that he and the
higher apes have evolved from a common distant ancestor;
they emphasize the similarities in anatomical structure, physiological characteristics, and behavioural patterns resulting
from this common ancestry. In contrast, sociologists and
humanists concentrate on the sociocultural aspects of human
life that set man apart from the rest of creation and even from
the higher apes. For sociologists and humanists, the significant
characteristics of man are those attributes and activities that
make him different from animals, not only in degree but essentially in kind.

When biologists state that evolution *transcended* itself in
producing man, they acknowledge their conceptual difficulties. Any attempt to demonstrate how typical human characteristics, such as the use of symbols and language or the
possession of consciousness and morality, can have originated
from an evolutionary transformation of purely biological
attributes meets with persistent rebuffs. To account for the

apparent discontinuity between man and animals, anthropologists postulated, in the 1920s, the 'critical point theory'. According to this theory – now out of favour – a sudden occurrence in the phylogeny of the primates gave early men the abilities required to develop a culture. The American anthropologist Alfred Kroeber taught that there had occured a critical mutation, probably affecting some limited part of the brain cortex and endowing a particular ape-man with the potential to generalize from isolated facts, to create symbols and thus to make him more efficient in learning from experience and in communicating his knowledge to the members of his group. According to this hypothesis, culture began with the activities of a newly endowed ape-man. Once begun, this culture, in theory, continued to develop progressively as a force independent of organic evolution.

Several lines of evidence suggest that the critical point theory is erroneous or at least grossly incomplete. The search for fossil remnants of man has yielded one of the strongest refutations. The discovery of a number of forms constituting a continuous series makes it impossible to draw a line between nonman and man on an anatomical basis. Since the bodies of hominids evolved progressively from an apelike nonhuman shape to that of modern man, probably the human mind evolved progressively also, rather than by a sudden mutation. Furthermore, the critical point theory of the emergence of culture was based on an assumption plausible at first sight but inconsistent with known facts. The assumption that the social aspects of human life began with *Homo sapiens*, the species to which we belong, contradicts all the modern evidence indicating that they were present in a rudimentary form in the precursors of man.

Until recently, anthropologists believed that physically and culturally primitive men created the first weapons and tools and established the rudiments of familial and social organization. These forerunners of modern men were presumed to be basically like us anatomically and mentally. Recent anthropological evidence strongly suggests that many characteristics regarded as typically human antedate *Homo sapiens* by several hundred thousand years. Human behaviour, it seems, emerged progressively from the ways of life of the precursors of man. So different were these early creatures from us not only in mental endowment, behaviour and social organization but also in structure that we would not claim them as fellow humans if they were existent today. In particular, the brain of these precursors of man was much smaller than our own.

It must be acknowledged that any statement concerning the emergence of man is at best speculative. Fossil remains of the precursors of *Homo sapiens* are so scarce and incomplete that imagination must often replace factual knowledge if we expect to link them into a continuous chain of descent. One thing at least is certain. Man did not originate from one of the higher apes that exist today; he is at the most one of their very distant cousins. As far as can be judged, the line of evolution from which man originated split from the proto-ape line far back in time during the Miocene period. From then on, unfortunately, a long period completely barren of firmly dated fossils ensues. Since as yet no precise biological definition of man exists, it is impossible on biological criteria alone to give even an approximate date for his emergence. The only recourse open is to identify manlike characteristics in prehistoric remains.

Some two million years ago, during the Pleistocene period, a kind of higher primate designated *Australopithecus*, but now extinct, lived in East Central and South Africa. This primate possessed a number of features suggesting humanization. Anthropologists consider that *Australopithecus* was sufficiently manlike to be classified as an early branch of the *Hominidae* rather than as a member of the *Pongidae*, the family of apes. Several types of australopithecines seem to have existed simultaneously; they differed in size and in minor traits, but all had a number of characteristics in common. The structure of their pelvic bones indicates that all of them could walk erect. Their canine teeth show a typically human reduction, suggesting that they were not used as extensively for cutting and tearing as in earlier evolutionary forms. The change in tooth structure may have been associated with a change in living habits, particularly with the use of tools. Crudely shaped tools estimated to be 1¾ million years old have been found in one of the famous Olduvai beds of East Africa close to fossils of *Australopithecus*. That the Olduvai bed also contains the remains of another form contemporary with *Australopithecus* somewhat obscures the significance of this finding, however. Physically somewhat more like modern man, this other form is designated *Homo habilis*. Several anthropologists doubt that *Australopithecus* was truly a direct ancestor of man and regard it rather as a sideline of evolution that eventually disappeared. *Homo habilis* may have progressively evolved into *Homo erectus* and then *Homo sapiens*. But this, too, is questionable.

Words such as *Australopithecus, Homo habilis* or *Homo erectus* are somewhat misleading because they imply well-defined species from which *Homo sapiens* descended in a direct line. In reality, the only certainty is that there existed during the Pleistocene period a multiplicity of higher primates, each sufficiently manlike to have been potential ancestors of *Homo sapiens*. Upright posture, bipedal gait, and the possibility of using the hands for manipulation are typically human characteristics apparently possessed by all of them. The point of emphasis here is that ape-men probably possessed the ability to make and manipulate primitive stone tools as early as two million years ago.

A substantial gap exists between fossils found in the Olduvai site of East Africa (the different types of *Australopithecus* and *Homo habilis*) and those of the various types collectively designated *Homo erectus* and generally, but not universally, regarded as direct ancestors of man. The difference is particularly striking with regard to the brain. The brain case capacity of the australopithecines was still within the ape range; moreover, the parietal and parietotemporal regions of their brains seem to have been poorly developed. Since these regions are the ones involved in the symbol-creating process, this finding is of special importance. The ability to symbolize is that quality most characteristic of man, since it has played the greatest role in the development of his cultures.

Several races of *Homo erectus* lived during the mid-Pleistocene period, approximately one million years ago Their fossils, found in different parts of Asia and probably also in Europe, have various designations such as *Pithecanthropus, Sinanthropus* and *Atlanthropus*. Uniformly they show larger brains and smaller teeth than those of *Australopithecus*. Even more important, the oldest evidence of the use and mastery of fire, probably man's first spectacular technological achievement, has been found associated with the remains of *Homo erectus* in China (Peking man). No fossil evidence exists for the transition between *Homo erectus* and *Homo sapiens*. Nevertheless, most students of early man believe that the line of descent was direct, even without knowledge of the steps leading from *Homo erectus* to true man.

Homo sapiens is first recognized on the Paleolithic scene in the form of the various Neanderthal races. One hundred thousand years ago Neanderthal men were distributed over much of western Europe and certainly extended as far as Palestine and Turkistan. They were on the average somewhat smaller than modern man, and they differed from him in a few other minor characteristics. Their foreheads were low, their frontal bone receding, and their brows heavy and protruding. Despite the shape of their skulls, their cranial capacity was very large for their body size, ranging from 1,300 to 1,600 millilitres in volume. Little is known of their way of life except that they buried their dead, evidence of some form of ultimate concern, unquestionably the most truly and mysteriously human characteristic of all.

The Cro-Magnon race of *Homo sapiens*, biologically identical with modern man, lived at the same time as the Neanderthal races. For reasons completely unknown, it either eliminated them or assimilated them by crossbreeding. Man with his present anatomical characteristics and mental endowment thus had become firmly established some 100,000 years ago, and from then on it is possible to speak of true human cultures. Various types of tools, many burial sites, artistic objects and other artifacts have been found in different parts of the world stages of the evolutionary process culminating in *Homo sapiens*.

While much remains to be learned concerning the final stages of the evolutionary process culminating in *Homo sapiens*, one generalization of great import has become increasingly apparent during the past few decades. Beginning perhaps with *Australopithecus* and almost certainly with *Homo erectus*, the hominids began to escape their animality and become humanized. This transformation thus began long before *Homo sapiens* had achieved the morphological appearance, particularly the brain size, characteristic of present-day man. Unquestionably, man was still evolving physically during the very period when he was developing the ways of life that would give rise to human cultures. As far as can be judged, his physical evolution was completed by the time the Upper Paleolithic bands of *Homo sapiens* had established the Cro-Magnon culture in Europe, approximately 35,000 years ago.

According to legend, Cro-Magnon man was a kind of superman, taller, better built and more noble than any people now living. While it is true that several disinterred skeletons of Cro-Magnon men suggest a height greater than six feet in the living specimen, such great stature was not the rule. Tall men may not have been more common among them than among us. What is certain is that the Cro-Magnon culture was highly developed. Cro-Magnon people buried their dead, at times in a crouching position and adorned with pigments and various artifacts. Some of their burial sites contain objects imported from long distances, an indication of well-established trade and commerce even at that early period.

A Russian report in 1965 revealed the discovery near Moscow of a 35,000-year-old skeleton dressed in trousers and pullover shirt made of fur and adorned with beads and a bracelet of mammoth ivory; the hands were resting together at the waist; the grave was stored with various kinds of tools. Unquestionably, therefore, Cro-Magnon man was preoccupied with the future and had achieved one of the attributes of modern man essential to the development of civilization. Numerous paintings, drawings, engravings and sculptures found in much of southern Europe and commonly known as cave art are usually attributed to Cro-Magnon man. If the attribution is correct, these artifacts prove the extraordinary extent of his artistic abilities and also strongly suggest that he participated in elaborate rites, further evidence of his concern with the future.

Fossil records indicate that, during the final stages of the evolution that produced *Homo sapiens*, extremely rapid changes occurred in the size of the parietal and parietotemporal region of the brain, changes simultaneous with more extensive use of weapons and other tools. Highly probable, but impossible to document adequately, is a contemporaneous increase in complexity of the ways of life, the social organization and the means of communication. In brief, it seems legitimate to assume that the evolution of the hand, the increase in the size and complexity of the brain, the diversification in the use of tools, the development of language and the spread of primitive culture all occurred during the same period and were influenced by each other.

Since many changes in man's nature and ways of life were simultaneous and interrelated, it seems worthwhile to speculate on the mechanisms of these interrelationships.

The act of childbirth may have played an extremely important role in the complex interplay between physical and cultural development. Man's acquired upright posture habit increased the difficulty of childbirth by changing the structure of the pelvis. In addition, language and culture created a selection pressure favouring a more complex brain and therefore a bigger head, rendering parturition more difficult. Probably a trend toward expelling the foetus somewhat earlier in its development resulted, and this in turn gave rise to a longer period of helpless infancy. Birth in an early phase of development is not peculiar to man. The marsupials are born the least mature of any mammals that bear living young. Also, the gestation period of man is longer than that of other primates. Relatively early birth has been of special importance for the social evolution of mankind, however, because it has exposed the human infant to the socializing influence of his mother and of his group precisely during his period of maximum plasticity. Under these favourable circumstances, human babies had an optimum opportunity for acquiring learned behaviour patterns. They could assimilate and later transmit the nongenetic, cultural heritage of the community. The need for more prolonged infant care may also have determined longer associations of the father with the mother and thus have contributed indirectly to the development of the familial and social structure.

The use of tools may be cited as an example of a cultural trait which had anatomical consequences. It seems reasonable to imagine that the first subhuman creature who picked up a stone and used it as a weapon or a tool perhaps opened an evolutionary channel; from that elementary start may have come the increasing ability to use weapons and tools and eventually to manufacture them, providing a selective advantage. The brain and language may thus have developed as a response to the invention and utilization of weapons and tools; these activities may have moulded both. Selection pressure provided the mechanism for guiding the incorporation of physical and mental skills in the genetic constitution.

Through analogous evolutionary feedback mechanisms, the development of family structure and of social practices for hunting in groups probably preceded somatic changes and the organization of reaction patterns. When early men began to supplement hunting small animals with big-game hunting, the greater complexity and magnitude of their group activities in planning and conducting the hunt required new attributes of leadership and new skills in communication. These social demands thus created a selection pressure for the development of new mental abilities. Soon after, perhaps, primitive forms of art and religion and systematic accumulation of experience and knowledge, the forerunner of science, also played their part in affecting the development of neural processes and their integration. Progressively, the most useful traits were selected for and embodied in the genetic code. New reaction patterns became moulded on the ways of life as the brain enlarged; reciprocally, the ways of life evolved as the brain and its functions became better fitted to them and more complex. At a late stage in the evolution of man, social mechanisms began to overtake genetic mechanisms in the transformation of human life. As we shall see later, this Lamarckian type of evolution is probably now more significant than Darwinian genetic evolution in the development of human societies.

The 'higher' functions of the human brain probably have their origin therefore in progressive structural-functional transformations from which developed a system permitting the physiological and behavioural adaptation of man to his own culture. By necessity, this adaptation cannot be perfect since culture is continuously being modified. What is almost certain, however, is that the various components of human culture are now required not only for the survival of man but also for the expression of his potentialities. Mankind emerged in the very process of creating culture and became dependent on the new world thereby created; the world of culture constituted from then on the natural environment of human life.

Fifty thousand years ago *Homo sapiens* was dispersed throughout most of the Eurasian subtropics and had even penetrated northward into the temperate parts of Europe and eastern Asia. Anatomical, physiological, and especially cultural adaptations enabled man for the first time to exist in regions with long and inclement winters. The modern races of man as we know them today with their characteristic body shape, skin colour and facial appearance probably represent late and secondary adaptations of *Homo sapiens* as he colonized the world at the end of the Glacial period.

The brain of modern man and his fundamental mental processes were certainly moulded early during the Ice Age, the formative influences being derived from the interplay between the culminating phases of his biological evolution and the

initial phases of his cultural development. These influences constitute, therefore, the common background out of which emerged the fundamental genetic makeup and cultural traditions of
mankind. Secondary adaptations producing the various human
races occurred only after the basic formative processes of
anatomical, neural and cultural development had been completed.

If this hypothesis is correct, it accounts for the remarkable
degree of biological and psychic uniformity throughout mankind despite environmental and social gaps separating the
races of man since Paleolithic times. It also explains why an
infant from a culturally backward people, adopted very early
in life by a more advanced cultural group, rapidly takes on the
behavioural characteristics of his foster society.

It will be recalled that one of the tenets of the ancient Great
Chain of Being concept was that no two varieties of life can
occupy the same place on the chain. Since human beings can
be divided into several races on the basis of obvious external
characteristics, it seemed necessary to allocate them different
places on the chain and therefore to rank them from the least
to the most noble, as was done for animals. Such a classifica-
tion of human races was taken for granted by most eighteenth-
century biologists, including the great classifier Linnaeus, and
many persons still widely accept it. Its persistence in that
form manifests itself in the public attitudes that are generating
the tragic events associated with the race problem all over the
world. But the biological concept of race, based on genetic and
biochemical distinctions, is a legitimate foundation for anthropological investigation.

Biological and Psychosocial Forces in Human Evolution

The more evolved an animal, the more unpredictable are its
behaviour patterns and its responses to environmental stimuli.
It is relatively easy to explain increased unpredictability in
species up to the lower mammals because greater freedom is
generally associated with the appearance of novel neural

mechanisms. It is more difficult to find in the anatomy of the brain a reason for the great degree of freedom exhibited by higher mammals, especially man. A profitable approach to the biological definition of *Homo sapiens* might therefore be to investiate the mechanisms through which man's evolutionary ancestors gradually attained more and more independence from external forces.

If present interpretation of anthropological findings can be trusted (a large if!), man had nearly completed his anatomical evolution some fifty thousand years ago; the human body and brain have remained essentially the same in structure and size ever since. In contrast, conditions of human life have changed profoundly during that period and continue to change at an accelerated rate. Thus two disparate phenomena, at first sight almost incompatible, must be reconciled in order to account for the biological history of the human race. On the one hand, the oragnic evolution of *Homo sapiens*, instrumented through genetic processes, has reached a near standstill. On the other hand, social evolution continues, almost independent of alterations in the genetic code.

The genetic stabilization of *Homo sapiens* is a phenomenon of such enormous importance that anthropologists have engaged in an orgy of imaginings to account for it. All of them agree that, as a result of the development of the brain, social mechanisms have now replaced genetic mechanisms as the most important aspects of human life. They also recognize unanimously how little opportunity presently exists for further organic evolution.

One of the most widely held theories traces the interruption of organic changes to the Late Paleolithic times when man became a hunter. The argument is based on the reasonable assumption that the men who were most alert became the leaders of hunting groups. These men achieved their dominance within the group through their ability to take aggressive, decisive action; concomitantly, they attained more ready access to the females, a pattern observed among primates living under natural conditions and among certain primitive peoples.

It is important to note in this regard that while the leaders in bands of primates living in their natural habitats are usually well endowed with certain kinds of 'mental' attributes, they are not necessarily the largest or most vigorous physically. Since what is true for primates today was probably true for early men, it can be assumed that the mental attributes associated with leadership acquired increasing importance with time and gave to their possessors a selective advantage in the reproductive pool. The practice of polygamy may have facilitated the genetic incorporation of these attributes into the tribe and may, in turn, have accelerated still further the evolutionary development of the brain.

The very increase of mental abilities within the group, so the argument continues, eventually led to a more complex social structure and, as a by-product, to a progressive replacement of polygamy by monogamy. When this social change occurred, it naturally reduced the rate of genetic evolution. Social institutions themselves assumed more importance than the attributes of individual leaders in providing the essential mechanisms of tribal activity. As a result, the leadership of the mentally gifted became less obvious, and their influence in selective reproduction consequently decreased.

Some anthropologists claim that polygamy and selection for enlarged brain size subsided as early as the Neanderthal stage. From then on, according to them, large-brained men no longer outbred their less brainy fellows. Other anthropologists dissent from this view and point to the continued prevalence of polygamy and the high fertility of leaders in certain contemporary populations. A recent report cites the example of a single Chavanté (Xavanté) Indian tribal chief in the Brazilian Mato Grosso who fathered one fourth of the hundred children in the next generation. The variety of opinions among specialists on this and related matters illustrates how much in the dark we still are concerning those selective factors that have operated in the past in bringing modern man's brain size and intelligence to their present levels.

Speculations concerning the origins of man and of his ways

of life cannot be supported by convincing evidence. Anthropologists, however, have no choice but to speculate in attempting to explain how biological mechanisms, as the main agency of change in human life, have been progressively replaced by social mechanisms. It will be noticed that the emphasis is on human *life* rather than on *man* himself. Changes in living conditions can and do rapidly bring about anatomical and physiological modifications and can even alter the genetic makeup of a population within a few generations. Witness the progressive disappearance of the sickle-cell gene among the Negroes living in North America or the spread of the porphyria gene among white people in South Africa. The point at issue here is that sociocultural forces are now vastly more important than the genetic ones in human *societies*. Herbert Spencer had such cultural forces in mind when he used the phrase 'superorganic evolution' to denote progressive changes in governments or banks and more generally in all social institutions.

Sir Julian Huxley, one of the grandsons of Thomas H. Huxley, the apostle of Darwinism in the nineteenth century, has repeatedly discussed the comparative roles of biological and psychosocial forces in the life of man. The following appropriate quotation, from a lecture delivered by Sir Julian in 1960 through the facilities of the British Broadcasting Corporation discusses the emergence of life and of mind as special manifestations of a more general cosmic evolutionary process.

We now believe with confidence, that the whole of reality is one gigantic process of evolution. This produces increased novelty and variety, and ever higher types of organization; in a few spots it has produced life; and, in a few of those spots of life, it has produced mind and consciousness.

This universal process is divisible into three phases or sectors, each with its own method of working, its own rate of change, and its own kind of results. Over most of the universe it is in the lifeless or inorganic phase. On earth (and undoubtedly on some planets of other suns) it is in the organic or biological phase. This works by natural selection and has produced a huge variety of animals and plants, some astonishingly high organizations (like our own bodies, or an ant colony), and the emergence of mind.

Finally man (and possibly a few other organisms elsewhere) has entered the human or, as we may call it, psychosocial phase, which is based on the accumulation of knowledge and organization of experience. It works chiefly by a conscious selection of ideas and aims, and produces extremely rapid change. Evolution in this phase is mainly cultural, not genetic; it is no longer focussed solely on survival, but is increasingly directed towards fulfilment and towards quality of achievement.[1]

The statement that 'the whole of reality is one gigantic process of evolution', as Huxley puts it, corresponds very closely to the evolutionary concept of creation ranging from matter to man and reaching to God, a concept formulated by the Jesuit Father Teilhard de Chardin two decades ago and delineated in his book *The Phenomenon of Man*. Sir Julian Huxley's warm introduction for Teilhard's book is therefore no surprise. In this introduction, he emphasized the ability of social man to rise within limits above the jurisdiction of natural selective forces and to gain thereby the power to govern his own evolution. Huxley expressed similar views during ceremonies in 1959 celebrating the centenary of the publication of Darwin's *Origin of Species*:

Man's acquisition of a second mechanism, over and above that of the chromosomes and genes, for securing both evolutionary continuity and evolutionary change, a mechanism based on his capacity for conceptual thought and symbolic language, enabled him to cross the barrier set by biological limitations and enter the virgin fields of psychosocial existence. ... Evolution in the psychosocial phase is primarily culture: it is predominantly manifested by changes in human cultures, not in human bodies or human gene complexes. (I am, of course, using culture in its broad anthropological and sociological sense, to include art and language, religion and social organization, as well as material culture.)[2]

1. René Dubos, *Torch of Life*, Simon Schuster, New York, 1962, pp. 77–8.
2. 'The Emergence of Darwinism', in Sol Tax (ed.), *Evolution After Darwin*, vol. I, University of Chicago Press, 1960, p. 19.

While most biologists agree with the general tone of Sir Julian Huxley's views, some of them question the wisdom of using the same word, evolution, to designate both the changes effected through genetic mechanisms and those brought about by social processes. Self-reproducing matter (biological evolution) and self-reproducing mind (cultural evolution) develop through such profoundly different mechanisms that each would seem to deserve its own terminology. According to present scientific usage, when the word evolution is used without further qualification by biologists, it refers exclusively to a Darwinian genetic process involving progressive alterations of the hereditary endowment embodied in the genes. In contrast, cultural evolution refers to all the facts and fancies, the rules and rites, the know-how and understanding that govern social life. The secular accumulation, modification and transmission of all these aspects of man's collective experience are mediated through social mechanisms that are increasingly independent of his genetic code.

Whatever the purists may say, the phrases psychosocial evolution and cultural evolution are now part of the scientific language even though they refer to mechanisms distinct from those operating in biological evolution. To complicate the problem further, some interdependence exists between biological and psychosocial evolution; these separate mechanisms of change are connected by feedback processes. When human societies alter their environment and their ways of life through cultural mechanisms, they create at the same time new conditions providing a selective advantage for certain biological characteristics of human beings. Psychosocial evolution proceeds to a large extent through nongenetic Lamarckian mechanisms, but it results almost inevitably in a certain amount of genetic Darwinian evolution.

So obvious are cultural forces in human activities that social scientists tend to believe that man has escaped from the clutches of biology. In reality, as we shall see later, biological forces still profoundly affect most of his individual and social life. Furthermore, some of the differences between exceptionally gifted persons and ordinary human beings certainly rest on a genetic basis. The thoughts and actions of a few exceptional persons have brought about most great advances in human history; their energies have given direction to the mass of the people. History is, in part at least, the outcome of forces set in motion by the peculiar genetic endowment of a few innovators.

Theoretical differences between the biological and psychosocial forces responsible for changes in human life have large practical implications. Changes mediated through genetic mechanisms are usually slow in manifesting themselves, but are lasting, and in many cases seemingly almost irreversible. In contrast, changes mediated through psychosocial mechanisms correspond to a Lamarckian type of evolution: the knowledge and skills acquired by one generation are transmitted directly to the next but persist only as long as conditions remain favourable for their direct transfer; what is gained through their agency in one generation can be completely lost in the next. History and everyday experience make it painfully clear that, under many trying circumstances, the primitive drives and urges of Paleolithic man readily break through the coating of civilization, precisely because civilized life arose largely from psychosocial changes rather than through organic evolution.

The Experiential and Social Past

All human beings have fundamentally the same anatomical structure, function through the same chemical activities, exhibit the same physiological manifestations, and are driven by the same biological urges. Yet, no two human beings are alike. Knowledge of the attributes shared by all mankind is therefore insufficient to account for the manner in which each person develops his own peculiarities and behaves as he does.

Except for the special case of identical offspring in multiple birth, individuals differ in their genetic makeup. At least equally important, the characteristics of individual human beings are constantly being moulded and altered by environmental factors. These factors endlessly vary with time, differ from one place to another and are never the same for any two different persons. Even identical twins fail to mature in close resemblance if each is raised in a different environment.

Recent studies have given substance to the ancient awareness that many characteristics of the adult human being result from the effects of 'early influences', those environmental factors impinging on the person while he is still developing. Such formative effects can take place even *in utero*. Although the Dionne quintuplets were genetically identical and were treated alike after birth, they could be recognized as individuals from the very beginning of their lives, probably because their positions during intrauterine life had differentially affected their development. Prenatal and early postnatal influences can affect almost every characteristic from nutritional needs and morphological appearance to learning ability and emotional attitudes. Moreover, the effects of early influences become so deeply rooted in the biological structure that they often and perhaps always persist throughout the whole lifespan.

Comparative anatomical studies of the various organs at different times after conception and after birth have done much to account for the profound, lasting, and often peculiar effects exerted by environmental factors on the developing organism. During the first two months of foetal life – the period of the embryo – the fertilized egg undergoes its most critical changes. Cells differentiate into specialized tissues such as muscle or nerve (histogenesis); the orginally homogeneous whole differentiates into specialized regions such as head or arms (regionalization); and at the same time each region is moulded into a definite shape (morphogenesis). Although the process of morphogenesis continues to adulthood, the major changes are completed during the first three months of intrauterine life. By then, the embryo has assumed a recognizable childlike appearance.

This simplified account of differentiation during embryonic

development helps to explain why nutritional deficiencies, exposure to toxic substances, and many other forms of stress experienced by the mother during the early stages of pregnancy so commonly cause birth defects and other abnormalities that become manifest only later in life. The early malformations in the foetus are rarely corrected during later stages of development.

Different tissues and different areas of the body grow at different rates throughout the formative period, prenatal or postnatal. This fact accounts for the changes that occur in body shape as development proceeds; it explains also why the response made by the various organs to environmental forces varies with their age. The development of the brain naturally presents a special interest in this regard because it has such direct relevance to the problems of learning and behaviour.

Early in foetal life the brain is nearer to its adult size in terms of gross weight than is any other organ of the body, except perhaps the eye. At birth the brain has reached about 25 per cent of its adult weight; at six months nearly 50 per cent; at five years 90 per cent; and at ten years 95 per cent. In this sense the brain develops earlier and faster than the rest of the body. Furthemore, the different parts of the brain do not develop simultaneously and do not grow at the same rate. Of greatest importance, the cortex has grown very little by the time of birth. Cortical structures and functions develop progressively, but many areas remain quite immature at two years of age, some retaining their immaturity until adolescence. During all the growth period, the number of dendrites increases, as does the probability of one brain cell influencing others through its connexions with them, a phenomenon referred to as 'connectivity'. When we realize that much of learning and of personality development occurs precisely at the time these connexions become established, we can understand the particular importance of connectivity.

During the brain's growth from its early foetal form to its conformation and capacity at two years, the development of function is closely related to maturation of structure, and this relationship probably continues throughout life. Experiments with rats have revealed that they are able to acquire certain behaviour patterns only when cerebral cortex connectivity reaches a certain level, irrespective of chronological age. There is good reason to believe that in man, also, the higher intellectual abilities appear when the maturation of certain structures or cell assemblies is complete throughout the cortex. Some neurologists believe that stimulation can influence brain maturation or organization, and that use of a cell can actually increase its connectivity. Underscoring this view is the observation that the first few weeks of life in the human species are spent largely in organizing perceptions, particularly the tactile and visual ones.

The likelihood that the mechanisms for perceiving and responding to stimuli are at least partly generated by earlier stimulation poses intriguing problems concerning the precise physicochemical reactions involved. Several such reactions have been postulated to account for the brain changes that result in learning and memory, but these hypotheses are at best highly speculative and no technique is yet available to determine their comparative merits. Definite physicochemical changes are known to be associated with learning, memory and other mental processes, however, and the time is near when the mechanisms of thought will become part of mechanistic biology as are the mechanisms of respiration or muscle contraction. Once knowledge has reached this stage, it is in grave danger of giving rise to a biomedical technology facilitating thought control for political and other purposes.

Educators could benefit greatly if they knew whether lack of stimulation retards or prevents neural organization, and how cell assemblies are affected by various influences exerted at different periods of life. Ideally, the manner of teaching and the times at which various things are taught should be governed by knowledge of the growth characteristics of the nervous system. Unfortunately, knowledge of brain development is still far from being sufficient to provide an effective guide for the formulation of educational programmes.

Evidence is conclusive, on the other hand, that neural development is affected by the nutritional state, by infectious processes, and by other environmental factors influencing health and disease. Thus, some of the largest problems of human development revolve around the physiological conditions of upbringing and the social environment, including all early influences and educational experiences. What effects they exert at different periods of life on the development of the brain determines their importance to human growth and behaviour.

The environmental influences that are ubiquitous in a given geographical area or social group naturally tend to bring out many characteristics common to all members of the group. For this reason there is much truth in Emerson's statement that 'Men resemble their contemporaries, even more than their progenitors.' Environmental influences also affect each person in an individual manner even when the ways of life appear uniform in a standardized environment. Genetic uniqueness makes for differences in response and, consequently, for singularities in mental and physical development. Each one of us lives, as it were, in a private world of his own.

Generally speaking, environmental influences shape personality through two different types of mechanisms. On the one hand, they determine certain patterns of response affecting all manifestations of behaviour. Physiologists, psychologists, psychiatrists and writers have described, each in his own way, a seemingly endless variety of acquired responses, ranging from the salivation of dogs at the sound of a bell to the pathological effects of the Freudian complexes, or the remembrance of things past evoked by a madeleine dipped into a cup of tea.

On the other hand, environmental influences contribute to the shaping of the personality by interfering with the acquisition of new experiences. In order to continue to develop mentally, ideally a person must remain receptive to new stimuli, new events and new situations. In actuality, however, the ability to apprehend the external world with freshness of *per-*

ception commonly decreases as the mind and the senses become conditioned by repeated experiences.

Human beings thus perceive the world, and respond to it, not through the whole spectrum of their genetic potentialities but only through the areas of this spectrum not blocked by inhibitory mechanisms and made functional by environmental influences, especially the early ones. The word potentiality here denotes the whole range of the organism's endowment, whether the characteristics it controls are physical or mental in nature. Life experiences determine what parts of this endowment become expressed in the form of functional attributes.

At the mature stages of life, traditional and conventional attitudes often interfere with the receptivity for new experiences, an inescapable result of early influences. By nature a child is playful and experimental. He is eager for experience and is constrained neither by conventions nor by inner conflicts. In contrast, an adult focuses his efforts on conscious and limited goals, narrowing the range of his receptivity to environmental stimuli. He practises selective inattention to those stimuli he assumes to be of no practical use and deliberately develops a kind of tunnel perception. Although permissible in navigating a route already determined, this attitude is ill suited to exploring new territory; almost invariably it tends to restrict the scope of life.

The tendency of the human personality to 'set' with age suggests some functional rigidification of the potential ability for continual progressive changes in the impressions stored in the brain, as if there were sharp limitations on what can be inscribed on the organism during its life-span. One of the great problems of biology is to determine whether the effects of early influences are truly irreversible, as ordinary experience seems to show, or whether they can be partially erased, as a few experiments suggest.

Electrophysiological studies have revealed that the activity of neural processes in the brain is continuous; the effect of stimuli is not so much to arouse inactive nervous tissue as to give form to the activity going on. Prolonged isolation and other forms of sensory deprivation are known often to result in a transient and more or less extensive breakdown of the personality. Taken together, these findings suggest that ways may be found to prevent or retard the 'setting' of personality so that man's body does not outlive the plasticity of his mental faculties. Tragically, brainwashing or induced confessions of political guilt and, more hopefully, certain forms of religious conversion supply the only practical evidence that the mind can be reshaped.

Loss of innocence during childhood is inevitable and is indeed a *sine qua non* of mental and emotional growth. What really matters, therefore, is the kind of experience through which innocence is lost, for this determines in large measure the characteristics of the adult personality. These characteristics in turn regulate the extent and direction of further growth.

Biological and psychological processes set in motion by interplay between human beings provide other examples of the lasting and profound influence of the past on modern man. Because he evolved as a social animal, man cannot develop well physically and mentally, or even long remain normal, unless he maintains close association with other human beings. Conversely, crowding and excess of social contacts may overstimulate certain of his hormonal activities and have undesirable consequences. The nature and intensity of the social stimuli that can safely impinge on the human organism have definite thresholds, but these thresholds differ according to the history of the person concerned and of his group. Qualitatively and quantitatively, man's responses to the social environment are conditioned not only by his genetic endowment and his early experiences but also by the traditional conventions and values of the groups within which he developed and in which he functions. Man's nature is inevitably conditioned by his social past. Usually man passively accepts the traditions of his group as embodying the truth; even when he rebels against them, the new traditions he tries to create always incorporate many of the ancient ways and continue to make him dependent on his social past.

The Uniqueness of Man

In the course of their evolution, the various animal species have developed a high degree of anatomical, physiological and behavioural specialization; as a result they have become committed to certain habitats and ways of life. Contrastingly, man has remained the great amateur of the living world. In many respects he is less gifted than other animal species now living. His vision does not reach into the ultraviolet as does that of the bees; his hearing, unlike that of dogs, cats and certain insects, does not extend into the higher ultrasonic range; his sense of smell is obviously inferior to that of dogs and other mammals. In brief, man is outdone by many animal species in such attributes as speed, physical strength, acuity of sense organs, accuracy of responses, and resistance to stresses. Probably he leads them all in adaptability, precisely because he exhibits so little biological specialization. In all likelihood, he has been able to undertake so many different kinds of tasks and to make his home in so many different parts of the earth by virtue of this adaptability.

The large size of his brain, particularly the development of his cerebral cortex, has been the essential factor enabling man to take advantage of his diversified biological potentialities. Comparison of animal species, including invertebrates, indicates that behavioural performance is correlated with the absolute size of the brain. While increase in brain size has been a notable feature of hominid evolution, the significance of actual brain volume in relation to mental functioning is by no means clear in modern man. True, some of the smallest brain sizes (below 1,300 millilitres) have been recorded for the Australian aborigines and other primitive peoples, but the range of cranial capacity is extremely wide and exhibits little if any relaton to intellectual ability. Probably more important than gross size in the mental superiority of man over animals has been the increase in higher, more recently evolved regions of his brain. These areas relate more directly to the development of culture.

In all higher animals the brain is the central organ of aware-ness. It has the amazing ability to integrate an enormous num-ber of separate and often disparate elements of experience into organized patterns. The organism as a whole is aware of each of these patterns and experiences each separately and distinctly from the rest. One of the most striking features of evolution is the gradual, progessive integration of all the cen-tres of 'mental' activity, a process that seems to have reached its peak in man. Certain areas of the human cortex specialize to some degree in the representation of sensory information from particular organs. Despite the relative independence of various channels of information and areas of representation, each person is convinced that he has one mind and not several and that this mind is ultimately the seat of all types of experi-ence.

Whatever the ultimate mechanisms involved, the most signi-ficant mental difference between man and animals is the much greater extent to which man can conceptualize. Probably of significance in this regard is man's early skill in making pic-tures; picture-making led to writing, an accomplishment en-abling him to transfer and perpetuate the impressions of his inner world.

As we have seen, animals demonstrate several levels of ele-mentary adaptive behaviour: simple conditioning, trial-and-error learning, and conscious, so-called insight learning, not apparently based on trial and error. All these various forms of learning occur naturally in man. In addition, man can call into play other learning processes either nonexistent or so poorly developed in animals that they cannot be recognized. Man can convert factual information into abstract ideas and words and later manipulate these mentally to create new types of be-haviour. He can elaborate abstract symbols and use them mentally in the absence of the original objects and percep-tions. The ability to conceptualize has helped him to acquire the kind of knowledge and adaptive behaviour he needed to master his environment.

Man's capacity to project his thoughts into the distant future, one of his most important attributes, gives him the motivating force to search for additional information and to make new efforts for types of learning leading to some distant goal. The human mind is hardly ever satisfied with existing situations and is always aspiring to higher achievements or to greater understanding. Ill-defined as it is, this aptitude for striving constitutes the dividing line between man and animals.

Certain social determinants of learning ability, recognizable among the higher primates, reach their highest level of development in man. Among the factors accentuating the role of learning in human social achievement are the biological tendency to bear only one or very few young and the long dependent growing period of man. The postnatal growth period increases from two years in lemurs to seven years in monkeys, to eleven years in the great apes, to approximately twenty years in modern man. This trend is associated with greater reliance on learned, as opposed to automatic, behaviours. Learned patterns of behaviour have the disadvantage usually of demanding a long apprenticeship, but they have the advantage of being more flexible and more adaptive.

The rearing process is probably most complex in *Homo sapiens*. Man's brain undergoes the greater part of its growth after birth. Whereas the ratio between adult and newborn brain weights in nonhuman primates is about 15 to 1, that for man is about 4 to 1. Even more impressive is the uncountable sprouting of dendrites and proliferation of synapses occurring after birth when the infant is exposed to the vicissitudes of the environment. It is therefore reasonable to assume that the structure of the human brain is largely determined by life experiences after birth.

Throughout the animal kingdom, adaptation has been achieved in the course of evolutionary development by an exquisite correspondence of the structures and reflexive behaviours of the organism to the details of its environment. Even very humble organisms also must learn about their environments and ways of life – the insect its leaf, the bird its song – but, on the whole, animal behaviour is largely innate and automatic. Such perfection, however, is gained at the cost of narrowing the range of adaptive possibilities; in addition, animals run great risk of inadaptation if the environment changes.

Man also has retained a number of behavioural automatisms as atavistic remnants, but he depends chiefly on learned behaviour. While the resulting range of potentialities is wider than that of any animal, the quality of the care he receives during early life profoundly affects their actualization. If care of the infant is mean and poor, the adult may achieve only a stunted expression of his potentialities, both in physical stature and mental development.

Language has long been thought to constitute the most absolute differential characteristic between man and beast, and experimentation lends credence to this commonsense view. Despite strenuous efforts, it has proved impossible to teach even chimpanzees to speak. It is not easy, however, to define with precision what is implied by the word language. Bees can communicate very precisely to other bees the location of distant food sources. Primates can warn their fellows of dangers and can apparently induce them to take certain courses of action. The fundamental difference may be that communication among animals does not deal either with the remote past or with the distant future; it does not extend to abstract concepts. As far as one can judge, it refers only to the here and now and the concrete.

The possession of language depends on the capacity for a varied combination of symbolic acts (sounds, gestures, writing). This ability developed in man along with greatly increased conceptual capacity through larger and more elaborate brains. This explanation, unfortunately, does not go much beyond stating that man has both a cerebral cortex more developed that than of other animals and the ability to speak.

It will suffice here to suggest that human language may not be unique in any particular feature. Its singularity may consist in the association and integration of several features that exist separately in various animal species.

Functionally, speech requires the activity of several areas of the brain to effect coordination between incoming and stored information and to achieve motor control of the muscular activities necessary for speaking. Since more than one area of the brain is involved in speech, the ability to speak cannot be diagnosed – contrary to a belief held in the past – from the enlargement of one of these areas as reflected in the endocranial cast. The study of fossils holds out little hope, therefore, of discovering definitely at which stage in evolution speech became part of the human endowment.

In any case, there is little doubt of the advantages conferred by the ability to speak. Although societies might exist without it, speech introduces much greater efficiency and versatility in all social functions. Many anthropologists believe that selection for speech was actually forced on the precursors of man by their increasing dependence on cooperative activities, especially by their need to transmit to other members of the group the knowledge necessary to make and use tools. Progress in the manufacture and use of tools depended on the development of language for communication, and language in turn became the crucial tool in the development of civilization.

The importance of the symbol system used in human language increases as the situation is removed from direct sensory or motor experience. Certain kinds of thinking related to social organization, morality or logic, for instance, could hardly be handled without symbolic language. It has been said that in most types of problems man can think only what he can say and that the categories of his language provide the categories of his perception, memory, metaphor and imagination. While this is probably an excessive statement, no doubt the ability to speak has been one of the decisive factors in shaping man's social and cultural behaviour. Furthermore, his use of a formalized system of symbols permits him to share otherwise private values dependent on memory, thought and feeling. Humanistic culture is hardly conceivable without language.

A generation ago, anthropologists were prone to define man as a primate who walks upright and has free forelimbs and hands. Benjamin Franklin's pithy words, 'Man is a tool-making animal', indicate that scholars of that time also knew man's attributes to involve more than bodily character. By now, however, it is recognized that tool-making is not a differentiating trait, since it is possessed by several species of animals. Nor can one define man by stating that he differs from animals because he knows how to design and use tools for a predetermined purpose. No matter by what single yardstick of ability one tries to differentiate man from animals – whether it be the power to communicate or to learn from experience or to act cooperatively, or even to engage in ideation and perhaps abstraction – one finds evidence of a similar capacity in other animals.

Yet it is obvious that man *is* different from other animals. Unfortunately, the only statement that can be documented objectively at present (which does not prove the validity of the statement) is that much of man's unique quality derives from a combination of characteristics all of which are found in other animal species, frequently only in an undeveloped state. A list of distinguishing traits present to some degree in higher animals but essential for the success of the human condition might read as follows: a superior degree of variability, erect posture, manipulative hands, an elaborate cerebral cortex, a prolonged period of immaturity and educability, skill in the use and invention of tools, symbolic speech and other communication systems, and the ability for conceptual thought and for art.

Food-sharing at home base, a highly organized and continuous family structure, rules of behaviour relating to incest and outbreeding, these are features of social life that appear to be almost exclusively human and to represent a sharp break between man and the higher primates. Although many men are grossly deficient in one or the other, mankind can go further and claim as peculiarly its own the acceptance of moral values that go beyond needs; a consciousness that transcends pure mentality; a conscience that overcomes fears; an interest in the remote past; and a concern for the distant future.

The concept of morality is perhaps more difficult to analyse and define than the ability to use symbolic language. It certainly involves empathic relationships to other human beings, complex attitudes that Martin Buber attempted to describe in the following words:

The inmost growth of the self is not accomplished, as people like to suppose today, in man's relation to himself, but in the relations between the one and the other, between men, that is, preeminently in the mutuality of the making present – in the making present of another self and in the knowledge that one is made present in his own self by the other – together with the mutuality of acceptance, affirmation and confirmation.

That the final stages of man's biological evolution occurred simultaneously with the initial stages of his culture makes it almost certain that biological and cultural characteristics cannot be considered separately. There is no such thing as a purely biological nature of man; it would be functionally unworkable. Tools, hunting and farming, familial and social structure, even religion, art and science all have played a part in the genetic moulding of man as we know him today. Because he evolves with his culture, man needs human culture for his survival and self-actualization just as much as he needs food and water. Culture patterns should not be regarded as external manifestations of man's nature. To paraphrase Clyde Kluckhohn, culture patterns constitute designs for human living.

Man is an animal, but an animal with immense ability to integrate all his sensations and perceptions into meaningful patterns. He is a reflective and interpretative animal, eager to find more than meets the eye in the bare data of experience. The reactions of his intellect combine with the brute facts of his sensible experience to enable him to manipulate the physical and social environment. The essence of his intellectual activity is to construct and utilize symbols as substitutes for the reality perceived by his senses. Man uses his intelligence to embody the experiences of life into his cultures and thus transmit them from generation to generation through social processes more rapid and more efficient than genetic mechanisms. He can produce new kinds of organizations of experience – scientific concepts, legal systems, moral codes, works of art – that constitute the building stones of psychosocial evolution.

The idea of self, conscious reflexion, and awareness that he is a mortal, these attributes have given to man a sense of history, a concern for the future. This concern has led him to develop a sense of values for his activities. His system of values expresses itself in the framing of conscious purposes with the hope that they can be translated into action. The belief that he *can* plan for the future and *should* indeed toil for a future transcending his own life-span is probably the ultimate manifestation of man's uniqueness.

Man Makes Himself

Biologically man has changed little since Late Paleolithic times. The implements he made during the Stone Age still fit our hands; the ancient drives that first shaped his tribal activities are still operative in us; the painting and sculptures of cave art and the artifacts symbolizing prehistoric beliefs still affect us emotionally. While *Homo sapiens* has remained essentially the same from the genetic point of view, the manifestations of his life and the structure of his societies are endlessly changing. The very concept of progress implies that events of human social life never repeat themselves identically. The permanency of man's nature resides in the chemical structure of his genetic code controlling the biological materials from which his body and brain are made; the change in man's life comes from the creative responses that he and his societies make to the challenges of the total environment. To live is to respond and thereby to activate the mechanisms responsible for adaptation and creative evolution.

Typical human urges, such as the need to play, are common attributes of animal life, and various types of social activity and organization – including their distorted pathological forms – characterize both natural and artificial animal communities. Students of human sexual behaviour can look for models not only in the monogamy of the gibbons but also in the permissive paternalism of gorillas, in the viciousness displayed in baboon harems, in the armed truce between chimpanzee males and females, as well as in the amiable polygamy of the New World monkeys and the sexual chaos of the rhesus monkeys.

Animals customarily resort to many 'typically human' behavioural manifestations, expressing their attitudes and desires through symbolic sounds, postures and objects. The male bowerbirds of Australia build elaborately decorated 'avenue bowers', love nests used not for egg-laying but designed strictly for luring females and for mating; the least handsome males build the most elaborate and colourful bowers, which constitute, as it were, a form of display to enhance their plumage. Kropotkin, in his book *Mutual Aid, a Factor of Evolution,* made clear that biological necessities often bring about social attitudes among animals, attitudes resembling human altruistic behaviour. No matter where one looks, one finds somewhere in the living world experimental models mimicking almost any aspect of human life.

While models are useful and essential tools in the scientific analysis of particular problems, they cannot provide a complete knowledge of man. Never truly representing nature, models illuminate only a circumscribed aspect of it. This limitation is not peculiar to the study of man or other living organisms; it applies to inanimate nature as well. Physicist Eugene P. Wigner made illuminating statements in this connexion in Stockholm on the occasion of his acceptance of the Nobel Prize for physics in 1963 :

... physics does not endeavour to explain nature. In fact, the great success of physics is due to a restriction of its objectives: it only endeavours to explain the regularities in the behaviour of objects. This renunciation of the broader aim, and the specification of the domain for which an explanation can be sought, now appears to us an obvious necessity. . . .

The regularities in the phenomena which physical science endeavours to uncover are called the laws of nature. The name is actually very appropriate. Just as legal laws regulate actions and behaviour under certain conditions but do not try to regulate all actions and behaviour, the laws of physics also determine the behaviour of its objects of interest only under certain well-defined conditions but leave much freedom otherwise.[3]

Freedom as used by the physicist when he refers to elementary particles has a meaning very different from the one it has when applied to human affairs. Nevertheless, the analogy, though only formal, helps explain why the biological information given in the preceding pages cannot give a full account of the living man whom the humanist tries to apprehend and the artist to express. Chemical biology can describe the materials from which man is made, but it does not explain how each person becomes what he is through a continuous series of accidents and personal decisions. A few remarks concerning the plastic arts will illustrate the manner in which man's ability to choose and to decide determines the limits of the relevance of biological knowledge to the understanding of man's nature. The paintings, statues, engravings and other artifacts found in Paleolithic sites leave no doubt that the faculty for artistic expression is very ancient. Neither in acuity of perception nor in representational skill has it shown marked improvement over the past twenty thousand years. Logic persuades us, therefore, that the ability to perceive and to represent corresponds to deep-seated physiological facets of man's nature.

The aesthetic faculty as it exists in man probably stems from biological attributes analogous to those that make animals perform movements or build nests of intrinsic harmony.

3. 'Events, Laws of Nature, and Invariance Principles', *Science*, vol. 145, no. 3636, 4 Sept. 1964, pp. 995–9.

All activities of animals and man are inevitably influenced by the innate periodicities that govern physiological processes and by the order prevailing in the patterns of the universe. Certain colours clash according to our vision, certain elements in a design appear to us out of proportion, when the experience of them conflicts with some built-in set of relationships in our organs or with the rhythms that we consciously or unconsciously apprehend in the external world. Conversely, we are displeased with the way certain things look, sound or feel unless our organs and senses are so constituted as to be in harmony with the proportions and rhythms associated with these things. Whether the satisfaction we derive when our senses or organs react to certain patterns and stimuli has a purely genetic basis or is the product of conditioning influences experienced in early life is irrelevant here. The point of importance is that aesthetic consciousness can emerge and flourish by virtue of innate faculties that are biological in essence and that do not seem to have changed significantly since Paleolithic times.

None of this implies that the ability to perceive and to represent is sufficient by itself to create human works of art; artistic creation involves factors outside the realm of the biological sciences. While human beings respond to their environment through their biological attributes, they do not react passively as if they were mechanical intermediaries in stimulus-response couplets. The artist's response is neither mechanical nor motivated by the desire to cope practically with the environment. His response constitutes rather an expressive behaviour; the artist uses his environment for self-actualization and at times to transcend himself.

The act of artistic creation thus provides a convenient illustration of the role of human choice in determining individual courses of action. Stimulated by his inherent needs, drives and urges, man can select from among the possibilities available for dealing with external nature. All aspects of human life present similar opportunities for active intervention on the part of man, the one creature who can consciously choose, eliminate, assemble and decide, and thereby move toward some selected goal beyond the here and now.

As knowledge of man's biological nature becomes more sophisticated, opportunities for the conscious manipulation of man's future open up. In a surprising but very real way, man becomes what he does. Through the complex feedbacks that govern all of life, man's biological endowment creates his culture and is in turn modified by his culture. Man is what he is today because he has been doing cultural and intellectual things for the past few millennia. The kind of creature he will become will be determined by the kind of activities he elects to emphasize in his life. Man is rapidly acquiring the technical knowledge that will enable him to manipulate his physiological and mental processes. Ultimately, he may even learn to manipulate his genetic makeup.

The power of action generated by recent scientific advances is so great that classical discussions on the ideals of the good life now take on unprecedented practical meaning. The ways in which human beings meet the dangers and exploit the opportunities of the modern world depend not only on the scientific knowledge and technology they possess but also on the beliefs they hold and the goals they select. The future of mankind rests on man's ability to make decisions based on ethical and aesthetic criteria.

We – that is to say, mankind – will drift aimlessly toward a state where we cannot maintain those values which make us unique among living forms unless we formulate goals worthy of the human condition and are willing to take a stand at the critical time. In the words of Paul Tillich, 'Man becomes truly human only at the moment of decision.' This kind of freedom is the final and finest criterion of humanness.

3 Biomedical Philosophies

The Human Past and Modern Medicine

Just as the long-domesticated dog still retains the fundamental characteristics of the wolf, so modern man retains many biological characteristics of his remote ancestors. Without question, the same set of genes that controlled the life of man when he was a Paleolithic hunter or a Neolithic farmer still determine his physiological needs and drives, his potentialities and limitations, his essential psychic and behavioural characteristics, and his responses to environmental stimuli. This evolutionary heritage combines with the experiences of his immediate past to determine his medical history and influence the medical problems he will face.

In order to analyse the effects of environmental factors on health and on disease, it is therefore necessary to keep in mind that man's life always involves a complex interplay between the conditions of the present and the attributes he has retained from his evolutionary and experiential past. A few examples will suffice to illustrate the extent to which the distant past still influences even the most purely biological aspects of modern human life.

Many important physiological functions of man exhibit diurnal, seasonal and lunar rhythms that persist even when a person is so completely shielded from changes in temperature and light that he is not aware of the movements of celestial bodies or of the passage of time. These rhythms were inscribed in man's genetic makeup at a time in evolutionary development when human life was closely linked to natural phenomena. The movements of the earth around the sun and of the moon around the earth are cosmic events unchanged since man acquired his fundamental characteristics. Even in his present artificial environment, biological rhythms persist in modern man. He may be unaware intellectually and socially of the diurnal, lunar and seasonal influences affecting his body, but he cannot escape the physiological and mental consequences of these cosmic forces. Some of his emotional states, too, may be related to the cosmic rhythms.

Primitive man also possessed automatic physiological mechanisms to enhance his chances for survival in the face of such threats as those coming from a wild beast or from a human stranger. These mechanisms rapidly mobilized in his body a number of hormonal and chemical reactions facilitating flight or fight, for safety or for victory. Today the so-called flight or fight response, in its many various forms, still comes into play when modern man finds himself in apparently threatening social situations. Stressful situations at the office or at a cocktail party elicit body responses similar to those occuring during a competitive sporting event or actual fight; these responses occur even though the need to expend physical energy rarely arises.

Physiological tests reveal that modern man has retained many such physiological and mental attributes ill suited to civilized life, just as he has retained useless anatomical vestiges from his evolutionary past. As a result, he must meet the challenges of today with biological equipment largely anachronistic. Many forms of organic and mental disease originate from the responses that man's Paleolithic nature makes to the conditions of modern life.

The Gods of Medicine

Like animals, primitive man had health instincts to help him overcome or minimize the effects of accidents or disease. In addition to these instincts, he must early have recognized some direct and obvious cause-and-effect relationships between certain empirical practices and the improvements of wounds or the alleviation of symptoms. Also, many forces he regarded as mysterious because they were indirect or outside the range of his conscious apprehension affected the health of primitive man. Magic thus early became an essential component of his attitude toward the causation and control of disease.

Medicine therefore had a dual nature from its very beginning. It included the empirical knowledge of effective procedures and belief in magical influences. Even today, medicine men in primitive populations supplement their practical skill in surgical technques and the use of drugs with a large variety of weird practices based on the tribal lore. Throughout history, and whatever the level of civilization, the structure of medicine has been determined not only by the state of science but also by the prevailing attitudes toward disease. These in turn are influenced by religious and philosophical beliefs. This is just as true of the most evolved urban and industrialized societies as it is of the most primitive populations. Like his Stone Age ancestors, modern man lives by myths.

With health and disease so inextricably related to every aspect of life, all ancient peoples have naturally given a prominent place in their theological systems to gods of medicine. Imhotep in Egypt, Shen Nung in China and Asclepius in Greece are but a few of the many gods of medicine whose names have come down to us and who are known to have inspired widespread cults thousands of years ago.

Ancient texts describe in detail the powers and virtues attributed by early civilizations to the various gods of medicine, and many documents describing them and their temples exist. Despite the abundance of information, it is extremely difficult to recapture the true medical significance of the knowledge and attitudes symbolized by the various deities. The Yellow Emperor's 'Classic of Internal Medicine', published in China several thousand years ago, asserts that health can be maintained through a way of life based on the doctrine of the *yin* and the *yang* and on respect for the laws of the seasons. Although modern scholarship has analysed at length these abstract principles of traditional Chinese medicine, their meaning remains obscure to us, so intimately interwoven is it with the philosophical subtleties of Chinese concepts of nature and existence. We cannot apprehend clearly how belief in the *yin* and the *yang* and in the laws of the seasons affected the professional activities of Chinese physicians or the expectations of their patients. We do not even know precisely how medieval mysticism or eighteenth-century rationalism affected the practice of medicine in Europe.

We can comprehend the thoughts and practices of physicians in classical Greece and Rome better than the doctrines of their Egyptian and Asian predecessors or contemporaries. At least we can legitimately claim to understand those aspects of Greco-Roman medicine surviving in our own medical culture. Like other ancient peoples, the Greeks traced the art of medicine to several different gods. Among them, Asclepius gained such prominence that his name became the symbol of the perfect physician. The Asclepian tradition is very ancient, complex and often obscure, but it encompasses several approaches to the problems of disease of significance to us because they have been incorporated in modern medicine.

During the classical period, the cult of Asclepius was under the control of a priesthood which practised faith-healing based on dreams. Drawn by a widespread and deep belief in the healing power of the god, many patients came to seek cures in sanctuaries dedicated to his worship but not organized for true medical care. These sanctuaries were built in beautiful surroundings, usually near a spring in the mountains or not far from the sea. Purifying baths, anointments, abstinence, a religious atmosphere, and the interpretation of dreams took the place of medical treatment in the temples of Asclepius. The immense number of offerings left by grateful patients healed in these temples – by the god, as they thought – is testimony to the effectiveness of faith-healing against certain diseases, especially when patients come to beautiful, healthy surroundings infused with a religious aura.

Faith healing as carried out in the temples did not, however, constitute the only form of the Asclepian tradition. Supposedly, Asclepius not only performed miracles but also knew the curative properties of drugs and was a master of surgical skills. Many lay physicians organized in medical guilds were trained in technical knowledge assumed to have originated with Asclepius. Called Asclepiads, these lay physicians nevertheless did not belong to the priesthood of Asclepius and had no connexion with temple medicine.

While acknowledging the healing powers of gods and goddesses, the lay Asclepiads practised a form of medicine based on the anatomical and physiological knowledge of their time and on the clinical experience acquired treating the sick. Probably they adapted a great portion of Mesopotamian and Egyptian medicine to the conditions of Greek life and thus acquired an extensive knowledge of surgery, drugs and regimens. As we shall see, the lay Asclepiad tradition, rather than the faith-healing performed in the temples, gave rise to Hippocratic medicine and indirectly to modern medicine.

Two goddesses, Hygieia (Health) and Panacea (All Heal or Cure All) represented the purely medical practices carried out by the lay Asclepiads. Both are often associated in classical iconography with Asclepius and are commonly described in Greek mythology as his daughters.

Hygieia was one of the manifestations of Athena, the goddess of reason. She was concerned not so much with the treatment of disease as with its prevention and with the maintenance of health. She symbolized the belief that men would remain healthy if they lived wisely, within the golden rule, and according to the laws of reason. *Mens sana in corpore sano* remains today the goal of all-embracing hygiene, even though men have found it difficult to do more than pay lip service to the teachings of Hygieia.

Panacea specialized in the knowledge of drugs. She symbolized the belief that ailments can be cured by skilful use of the proper kinds of substances derived either from plants or from the earth. The illusion that drugs can solve all medical problems survives today in our use of the word 'panacea'.

Hygieia and Panacea, along with Asclepius, were specifically mentioned in the opening invocation of the Hippocratic Oath taken by physicians when they were admitted to the Asclepiad guild. The association of the three deities in the oath indicates that ancient physicians differentiated between prevention and treatment of disease and recognized the importance of both types of medical activity. Greek legend thus anticipated some of the most important theoretical attitudes of modern medicine.

Hygieia and Panacea symbolize two radically different yet complementary approaches to the control of disease. These two attitudes have their counterparts in all great cultures, particularly in the Judaeo-Christian tradition. in the Old Testament, the ancient Hebrews codified many precepts of behaviour based on sanitation and on purity in all its forms, physical and mental. These precepts certainly contributed to the control of crowd diseases as well as to the maintenance of individual health. The tradition of succouring the sick and bringing them back to health also has deep roots in the Old Testament. Hebrew precepts eventually were identified with Christ, the Healer, and later assimilated the Asclepian beliefs and practices which had spread from Greece to the whole Mediterranean world. A beautiful marble head of Christ, adapted from a bust of Asclepius, found in Palestine, symbolizes the merger of the Greek and Christian healing traditions. As in Greece, dreams played a large part in the miracles performed by Christian healers, particularly by Cosmas and Damian, the two saints identified with medicine and pharmacy.

The legendary attributes of the ancient gods of health and medicine appear at first sight completely unrelated to the scientific concepts and practical achievements of modern medicine. When we reflect that our world has two different kinds of medical establishments corresponding to the two general methods of disease control symbolized in the Greco-Roman world by Hygieia and Panacea, we can understand the relevance of the ancient medical tradition. The schools of hygiene (or public health) emphasize the *prevention* of disease in the community as a whole through healthy social practices.

The schools of medicine are primarily concerned with the *treatment* of disease and with the care of individual patients. Like Asclepius, a modern physician needs the knowledge of these two sister branches of medicine. He must teach ways of life and sanitary practices that minimize the occurrence of disease. He must also help stricken persons by any means at his disposal. In the performance of his profession, he must not only use drugs and surgery but also exert psychic influences not far removed from the health-restoring practices which benefited so many patients in the Greek temples of Asclepius.

The Hippocratic Tradition

In all the countries of Western civilization, physicians recite the Hippocratic Oath, or a modification of it, either when they graduate from medical school or during the ceremonies of initiation into learned medical societies. This gesture implies allegiance to the high ethical principles inherited by the medical profession from its distant past. It constitutes also a tacit acknowledgment of the profound influence of Hippocratic doctrines on the development of Western medicine.

Nothing is known of Hippocrates the man except that a famous physician by that name lived around 400 B.C. on the Greek island of Cos where he practised and taught medicine as a lay Asclepiad. Although the several books attributed to Hippocrates are quoted so frequently and with such respect that together they are almost the equivalent of a medical Bible, we have no valid historical information concerning their real authorship. The various parts of the *Hippocratic Collection* contain many differences in style and contradictions in medical doctrine, sound evidence that the texts collected under this name were written at different times, in different places and by different authors. The consensus now is that the so-called Hippocratic writings represent a compendium of the medical knowledge shared by the members of various Asclepiad guilds. The texts were probably assembled into a unified body of teaching by the Alexandrian scholars of the third century.

The fundamental philosophy of Hippocratic medicine is that diseases are not caused by capricious gods or irrational forces, as primitive people are wont to believe. They constitute natural phenomena developing in accordance with natural laws. Disturbances of the body and the mind can therefore be studied just as objectively as any other natural phenomenon; they can be understood by reason and controlled by the wise management of human life. Hippocratic philosophy contends that medicine is not an appendage to religion; it can and should be practised as a true scientific discipline. Commonplace as this attitude appears today, it developed slowly and has yet to be adopted universally. Even partial acceptance of the Hippocratic doctrines has led, nevertheless, to the formulation of a number of principles shaping the theory and practice of modern medicine.

The primary Hippocratic principle is that medicine should be based on the natural sciences. The physician should have profound knowledge of the biological phenomena of life in health and in disease; he should be able to recognize the logical relations between cause and effect. According to the Hippocratic doctrines, this scientific approach leads to the following conclusions:

1. The well-being of man is influenced by all environmental factors: the quality of the air, water and food; the winds and the topography of the land; and the general living habits. Understanding the effects of environmental forces on man is thus the fundamental basis of the physician's art.

2. Health is the expression of harmony among the environment, the ways of life, and the various components of man's nature. For the Greco-Roman physicians, four humours determined man's nature: the relationship between blood, phlegm, yellow bile and black bile controlled all human activities.

3. Whatever happens in the mind influences the body and the body has a like influence on the mind. Mind and body

cannot be considered independently of each other. Health means therefore a healthy mind in a healthy body. It can be achieved only by governing all activities of life in accordance with natural laws so as to create an equilibrium between the forces of the organism and those of the environment.

4. Whenever the equilibrium is disturbed, rational therapeutic procedures should be used to restore it by correcting the ill effects of natural forces; these procedures should include the use of regimens, drugs and surgical techniques.

5. The practice of medicine implies an attitude of reverence for the human condition and must be based on a strict code of ethics.

Paraphrasing Whitehead's remark on the debt of European philosophy to Plato, one can state with much justification that modern medicine is but a series of commentaries and elaborations on the Hippocratic writings. By their comprehensive coverage and their depth of understanding they have retained a universal appeal into our day. The scientist recognizes in them the first known systematic attempt to explain the phenomena of disease in terms of natural laws; he shares the interest of the Greek physicians in precise observations objectively made and carefully recorded. The clinician admires Hippocrates for his shrewd observation of signs and symptoms characteristic of each disease, for his knowledge of prognosis based on clinical experience, and for his penetrating concern with the patient as a complex human being integrated in his community. The student of public health points to Hippocratic emphasis on the roles of environment and ways of life in the occurrence of disease. The student of man's natural history is impressed by the statement in *Airs, Waters and Places* – one of the most searching books of the *Hippocratic Collection* – that the general characteristics of human populations in the normal state are conditioned by the topographic and climatic factors of the locality. Much of modern medicine consists in the unfolding and elaboration of Hippocratic concepts.

The Body Machine

Practising physicians have always known that the various aspects of human life are closely interdependent and that effective care of the body demands attention to the mind,[1] and the reverse. Medical scientists also are interested in the whole man, but they know from experience that to apply the scientific method to the study of human problems they must first artificially simplify them. In practice, the various components of man's nature must be studied either separately as independent structures and functions or in arbitrarily simplified combinations.

René Descartes and his followers introduced the most far-reaching scientific simplification of the study of man in health and in disease. Descartes predicated the assumption that man consists of two separate entities, body and mind, linked during life but profoundly different in kind. He claimed that since the mind is a direct expression of God its nature cannot be understood by science. In contrast, he taught that the body is a machine whose structure and operations fall within the province of human knowledge. Many scientists, philosophers and theologians question the validity of the body-mind dualism concept, but no one doubts that Descartes' philosophy has exerted an immense influence on the evolution of biological sciences in general, particularly in medicine.

Whatever its philosophical limitations, the concept of body-mind dualism has proven operationally useful; it has helped

1. Many scholars object to the use of words such as 'mind' or 'mental' because these do not refer to well-defined attributes. They find no justification in particular for using the word 'mind' as a noun, and they urge that it be restricted to its grammatical function as a verb. According to many psychiatrists and experimental psychologists, it is correct to say 'mind the baby' or 'mind your own business', but not 'he has a fine mind' or 'his mind is deranged'. Admittedly, there is no evidence that 'mind' refers to a location, a structure, or a substance in the body. In practice, however, even the most materialistic philosopher has no doubt that his own 'mind' is better than that of the village fool. For reasons of convenience, we shall therefore continue here to use the word 'mind' as a noun, even without convincing knowledge of the structures and processes thereby implied.

scientists to delineate more precisely the scope of their investigations. Instead of attempting the hopeless task of understanding man as a whole, scientists have felt free to deal *seriatim* with the various aspects of man's nature.

Descartes' philosophy led scientists to neglect questions pertaining to the nature of the mind and the soul and encouraged them to focus their efforts on the much simpler, more concrete, problems of body structure and operation. They could apply knowledge of physics and chemistry, derived from the study of inanimate matter, to the problems of the body without fear of debasing the more lofty manifestations of man's nature, those of his soul. The self-imposed limitations and the intellectual freedom that biologists derived from Cartesian dualism gave them a general tendency to study man as a nonthinking, nonfeeling entity.

Since Descartes' time, the study of the body machine, its structure and its functions, has reflected directly the state of knowledge in physics, chemistry and other natural sciences. At first, scientists delighted in describing and measuring the mechanical aspects of the body; they built mechanical contrivances in the image of animals and human beings, machines capable of performing complex manoeuvres. During the nineteenth and twentieth centuries the emphasis shifted to the chemical interpretation of living processes. Physiologists became impressed by the resemblance between bodily operations and those in a factory; as a result, the physicochemical problems of nutrition, metabolism and energy requirements have been foremost in the study of man.

The physicochemical analysis of life has progressed so far that the fabric and the functions of the human body can now be described in precise laboratory language. Molecular biology can provide approximate pictures of the giant molecules constituting the most essential parts of the body and of the chemical reactions that keep it functioning. The nucleic acids and their associated proteins have been shown, furthermore, to act as information-carrying systems, transmitting hereditary characteristics from one generation to the next and integrating the multifarious activities of the organism. Even the brain is being described in physicochemical terms. Increasing knowledge of feedbacks and of servomechanisms has revealed that mental activities exhibit some of the characteristics of complex electronic computers.

René Descartes pictured the nervous system as a complicated hydrostatic system of hollow tubes conducting animal spirits to and from the brain. Charles Sherrington borrowed models from early twentieth-century physics and electricity for his classical analysis of spinal-reflex mechanisms. F. R. Lillie compared the events in nerve conduction to those of an iron wire bathed in acid and coated with a salt. More recently, many operations of the brain have been compared to the workings of an electronic computer that can 'learn', 'remember' and 'make decisions'. In the words of the English physiologist J. Z. Young, 'The brain can be regarded as an exploratory, self-instructing computer that acts as a controller of the homeostat represented by the organism.'

Biological science is continuing to develop along the channels first opened during Descartes' time. From contrivances imitating the mechanical motions of the body, biologists have moved to models representing the genetic code and to electronic problem-solving machines that learn from experience. This trend in biology has carried over to other aspects of medical science. When a physician wants to become a scientist, he is prone to act as a Cartesian. He studies not the whole man but either the body or the mind and usually limits himself to even narrower aspects of man's total nature.

Modern physicochemical knowledge of the structures and mechanisms through which the body machine operates has facilitated diagnosis and treatment of disease. The development of new medical procedures is now so dependent on general biology, chemistry and physics that a more extensive application of these sciences to the study of living things is a *sine qua non* of medical progress. The practical problems posed by the prevention and treatment of disease, however, involve many factors other than those encompassed within the present physiocochemical formulation of the body machine.

Though Descartes' philosophy of body-mind dualism provided a favourable environment for the emergence of the modern biomedical sciences, the validity of the philosophy itself is open to question. Many medical scientists believe that Cartesian dualism, useful as it has been, is leading medicine into a blind alley precisely because it is philosophically unsound. They contend that the processes of the 'mind' are not different in principle from those of the 'body' but are merely less understood because of their complexity. Presently, great efforts are being made to apply the methods of the natural sciences to the problems of the mind. These efforts can be classified in two general groups. Some investigators are following what might be called the 'components' approach. They use the analytical methods of biochemistry, biophysics and molecular neurology to determine the intimate structures and mechanisms involved in such processes and attributes of the 'mind' as learning and memory. Others follow the 'systems' approach and use the more functional procedures of neurophysiology, psychology and the social sciences. The components approach leads to a detailed knowledge of the brain, whereas the systems approach is more concerned with the functions referred to by the word 'mind'.

These efforts to account for the operations going on in the brain have produced some new, exciting theories. Experience shows that most physicians, however, irrespective of their professional activities and philosophical views on the nature of the mind, behave in practice as if they were still Cartesian dualists. Their conservative attitudes are largely a matter of practical convenience. So far, the knowledge acquired by studying the brain with the techniques of the physicochemical sciences has not contributed significantly to an understanding of the mind's processes and their relation to the body mechanisms. From the pragmatic point of view, it is still usually more useful to think of the mind as a distinct attribute of life associated with the body as long as consciousness lasts but different from it in practical manifestations. Since the welfare of the body and of the mind are differently affected by various factors in the environment, the tendency on the part of physicians to separate the two is understandable. Conditions for mental misery may be compatible with glowing physical health, and happiness may reside in a diseased body.

The only safe generalization at the present time is that the body and the mind constantly interact and constitute an integrated whole. Furthermore, all the problems of health and disease are the expressions of the effects of the environment on the genetic apparatus. Today, as in Hippocrates' time, good medical care implies attention not only to the body but to the whole person and to his total environment. In this light it seems appropriate to consider briefly some of the present medical attitudes concerning the body-mind-environment interplay, even though no final statement can be made concerning the nature of the mind itself.

The Whole Man

All natural phenomena are the result of complex interrelationships; all manifestations of human disease are the consequence of the interplay between body, mind and environment. This situation creates a difficult dilemma for physicians and medical scientists. They recognize that the analytic breakdown of the problems of disease into their component parts never results in a true picture; yet they know from practical experience that the artificial reduction of these problems into their constituent parts, or their conversion into simpler models, is an absolute necessity for scientific progress.

The operations of the mind provide particularly striking examples of the need for artificial simplification in biomedical research. Even the most casual observer can see from daily life that the condition of the body affects mental processes, and that, reciprocally, our state of mind affects most organic processes. In practice, problems of the mind have been the specialized province of experts who tend to remain aloof from the problems of the body. These experts have been subdivided into several groups hardly in communication with each other. Depending upon their scientific philosophy, the different schools of psychologists and psychiatrists have looked at the mind, each from a different point of view. All have been affected by the social and religious doctrines prevailing in their communities.

Frequently in the ancient world mentally deranged people were assumed to be in contact with supernatural forces and were believed to be endowed with superior, extraordinary powers. Insanity was often revered as a gift for prophecy. Later, the belief developed that insanity was caused by demonic possession and could be cured only by exorcising the devil and other demons from the demented person. As time went on, insane people came to be regarded not as true human beings but as sinful and subhuman creatures; in consequence, they were removed from normal society and held in chains like savage beasts. Surprising as it may seem to us, this attitude prevailed in the most civilized countries of Europe during the eighteenth century, and it persisted until the early part of the nineteenth century. As late as 1805 the Scottish anatomist and neurologist Charles Bell asserted that insanity was the result of sin. In his famous textbook, *The Anatomy and Philosophy of Expression*, he stated explicitly, 'If madness is to be represented, it is with a moral aim, to shew the consequences of vice and the indulgence of passion.' He illustrated this statement with a drawing of a beast-like madman restrained in chains.

Social and scientific attitudes concerning mental diseases began to change one hundred and fifty years ago when humanitarianism and respect for the individual emerged as dominant social philosophies. A few humanitarian laymen and physicians suggested that insanity was not the result of sin or demonic possession but a human tragedy caused by the accidents of life. They concluded that chaining insane people and beating them into submission was social immorality as well as bad medicine. As a substitute they advocated the removal of the noxious environmental influences that injure people mentally, and they suggested therapeutic methods to restore to normal life persons suffering from mental disorders.

Rejection of the demonic theory made it possible to regard mental diseases as natural phenomena amenable to objective scientific study. This change of attitude soon found expression in a many-pronged analysis of the nervous system and the mind, its goal a better understanding of the mechanisms of mental processes and of the disorders leading to aberrations of behaviour. If we glance briefly at two of the varied scientific approaches to the problems of the mind, we can grasp how essential, though intellectually objectionable, is the narrowing of interests to the growth of knowledge and how compatible it is with a holistic view of body-mind relationships.

Ivan Pavlov's celebrated experiments at the beginning of the twentieth century on conditioned reflexes constituted the earliest systematic investigations of biological mechanisms involved in mental processes. These experiments followed and were closely linked to earlier studies on the physiology of digestion. His observation of dogs used in physiological studies convinced Pavlov that a complete understanding of digestive processes required a deeper knowledge of neural mechanisms controlling the secretion of digestive juices. This concern led him to recognize the importance of conditioned reflexes and to analyse their neurological determinants.

Although Pavlov's fame rests largely on the relevance of his neurological discoveries to the various forms of behaviourism, he never lost sight of the intimate relationships existing between neural phenomena and organic processes; this awareness is evidenced by his systematic use of a purely physiological operation, salivary secretion, for measuring a neural one, reflex activity. Ironically, the various schools of psychology and psychiatry that derive their inspiration from Pavlov's work hardly ever trace the origin of his influence to his purely physiological studies of digestion.

Sigmund Freud, the other towering historical figure in the study of the mind, also was originally concerned with the interrelationships between mental and organic processes. His first investigations dealt with the physiological effects of drugs on certain mental states. As a result of observations on hypnotic states and the development of the psychoanalytic method, Freud, and more so his followers, abandoned these early physiological preoccupations. Freud himself did not forget the physiological origin of his studies; late in life he expressed his conviction that the 'complexes' he had described in purely psychiatric terms would one day be traced to faulty organic processes. The psychoanalytic schools, however, have evolved almost independent of the physiological sciences and of other fields of biomedical knowledge.

As mentioned earlier, scientists and physicians may question the philosophical validity of Cartesian dualism, but in practice they usually act as if the mind and the body were either distinct in their natures or in their manifestations. They therefore approach the study of the mind with techniques quite different from those they advocate for the study of the body.

Unquestionably, the psychoanalytic schools sharpened physicians' awareness of the interplay between mental and bodily functions. One of the important advances of twentieth-century medical science is the recognition that many kinds of stimuli, especially those experienced in early life, can affect not only psychic reactions but also organic processes. The body and the mind are thus seen to be affected by the same conditioning factors. From this new awareness came the development of an intellectual atmosphere unfavourable to Cartesian dualism.

Psychosomatic medicine, concerned primarily with the causation of organic disease by mental disturbances, was an outgrowth of the enlargement of thought brought about by the Freudian revolution. It found its intellectual support among those dissatisfied with the narrow application of Cartesian dualism to medical problems; it received public support from the awakening recognition that much organic disease obviously has its origin in emotional states. Many physicians, however, have now gone still further toward identifying the organic and mental aspects of disease and deny the need for a psychosomatic theory of medicine. It is now realized that pathological conditions usually have both somatic and psychic components in their causation and in their effects. Physicians' observation that almost anything happening in the mind affects the operations of the body, and vice versa, makes it misleading to single out certain diseases as having a psychosomatic origin. Whatever its precipitating cause and its manifestations, almost every disease involves both the body and the mind, and these two aspects are so interrelated that they cannot be separated one from the other.

The understanding and control of disease requires that the body-mind complex be studied in its relations to external environment. Most immediate medical problems have their origin in the responses of the human organism to present environmental forces.

The study of these responses became a dominant theme of biomedical science after Claude Bernard pointed out that the internal environment of the healthy human organism remains essentially constant even when the external environment fluctuates widely. The recognition of the constancy of the internal environment constitutes such an important landmark in the emergence of modern medical philosophy that physiologists are prone to use the French expression *milieu intérieur* when they want to refer to the internal environment. They acknowledge thereby the importance of Claude Bernard's famous dictum: *La fixité milieu intérieur est la condition essentielle de la vie libre.* ('The constancy of the internal environment is the essential condition of independent life.') Much of physiological science during the past one hundred years has been concerned with the analysis of detailed mechanisms through which the body attempts to maintain the constancy of its *milieu intérieur*.

Around the turn of the century, W. B. Cannon enlarged Bernard's concept by directing attention to the hormonal mechanisms that come into play whenever the body responds to environmental stimuli. He recognized that when these stimuli bring about transient departures from an ideal state the hormones and other physiological agencies act as regulatory mechanisms and tend to correct disruption in the internal environment. They maintain what Cannon called a state of homeostasis or a relative stability of body functions.

Homeostasis implies two separate, but interdependent, concepts. One recognizes that the body can function well only if its *milieu intérieur* remains within limits characteristic for each organism. The other acknowledges that the body must make rapid adjustments to correct for the disturbing effects of constantly changing external conditions. In principle, health can be maintained only if these two conditions are simultaneously satisfied through complex hormonal and biochemical processes governed by what Cannon picturesquely called the 'wisdom of the body'.

Like the constancy of the *milieu intérieur*, homeostasis is a concept of the ideal. Living organisms do not always return to the exact former state following a disturbance by an environmental stimulus. The organism's response often fails to re-establish the original *milieu intérieur*, and in many cases, the response is not even appropriate to the welfare of the organism. It may be excessive or misdirected and result in injurious or destructive reactions. Disease is commonly the consequence of such inappropriate responses.

While Bernard and Cannon were chiefly concerned with the governing role of biochemical and hormonal reactions in the maintenance of homeostasis, the Russian school began very early to focus its attention on the part played by neural mechanisms in the control of responses to environmental stimuli. Among the first to emphasize that body processes are subject to regulation by neural integrative mechanisms were I. M. Sechenov and S P. Botkin; their teaching created a favourable intellectual atmosphere for Pavlov's studies of the influence that the cerebral cortex exerts on visceral functions.

In the normal organism, neural reactions integrated at the highest level do govern man's responses to physical or mental stimuli. Ideally the reactions originating in the cerebral cortex protect the organism against damage, or facilitate its adaptation to the environment. Unfortunately, the physiological responses set in motion by the neural mechanisms often take the form of inflammatory processes or other highly destructive tissue reactions. The so-called adaptive response can be misdirected also in the case of mental stimuli. Although psychologists are prone to state that most behavioural manifestations are adaptive in goal, all too often the effort at adaptation results in a neurosis that is mentally incapacitating. In its mental as well as in its physical manifestations, the wisdom of the body is thus far from perfect; the ultimate results of seemingly protective or adaptive responses sometimes turn out to be deleterious.

Most of the great achievements of modern medical science have been in fields having to do with the disorders of the body machine. To a much more limited extent, some independent progress has been made toward understanding and controlling behavioural abnormalities. The need for a theory linking these two fields of medicine becomes more and more urgent as clinical experiences reveals that many, and perhaps all, disease states are the expressions of both organic and psychic factors.

Clinical and epidemiological studies show that the inextricably interrelated body, mind and environment must be considered together in any medical situation whether it involves a single patient or a whole community. In a long, roundabout way, scientific medicine is thus returning to the unitarian concept of disease intuitively perceived by the Hippocratic physicians two and a half thousand years ago. Whatever the complaints of the patient and the signs or symptoms he manifests, whatever the medical problems of the community, disease cannot be understood or successfully controlled without considering man in his total environment.

The holistic approach, however, corresponds to an abstract ideal not amenable to full achievement in practice either by the clinician or the public health officer. Most medical situations are so complex that their determinants can never be apprehended in all their details; it is impossible consequently to deal with them only on the basis of scientific knowledge. While it is philosophically correct and intellectually appealing to think of the whole man in his total environment, this holistic attitude rarely lends itself to the acquisition of precise knowledge.

Scientists realize that the reductionist analysis of the body machine and of its functions cannot provide a complete understanding of human problems, but they are willing to accept that medical science must work within certain limitations, at least for the time being. They leave to practising physicians the responsibility of integrating the isolated fragments of knowledge and of applying these as best they can to the complex and often ill-defined medical problems of living persons. To approach the ideal, precise scientific knowledge of the body machine must be supplemented with a more empirical attitude in the practice of medicine.

Whether a particular problem concerns the care of an individual patient or the formulation of public health policies for large numbers of people, the art of medicine consists to a large extent in the ability of medical men to devise practical measures best suited to the human beings involved. Usually, physicians must deal with problems they cannot fully comprehend and conditions that they cannot entirely control.

Objective knowledge somewhat different from that derived from the reductionist analysis of the body machine is needed to provide a broader and more secure scientific basis for the art of medicine.

4 Determinants of Health and Disease

Health and Disease Defined

The difficulty of defining disease is implied in the very structure of the word: 'dis-ease'. So many different kinds of disturbances can make a person feel not at ease and lead him to seek the aid of a physician that the word ought to encompass most of the difficulties inherent in the human condition. Generally, especially among the lay public, disease implies some serious organic or psychic malady such as cancer or insanity. Modern medicine in practice is broadening this concept to refer to any state, organic or psychic, real or imaginary, that disturbs a person's sense of well-being. In this sense, disease may threaten life or simply interfere with its enjoyment; it may prevent the sick person from functioning as a normal human being or simply from reaching his self-selected goals. Physicians now realize that in dealing with the problems of the 'dis-eased' person subjective and social factors may be as important as the objective organic lesions or behavioural disturbances recognized by the pathologist or the psychiatrist.

It seems reasonable at first sight to define health as the absence of disease. This definition falters in the very uncertainties and complexities referred to in the preceding paragraph. The all-inclusive and consequently vague meaning of the word health can be traced all the way back to its Anglo-Saxon root, which means 'hale', 'sound', 'whole'. Irrespective of precise medical criteria, the experience of feeling healthy has always consisted in being able to function well physically and mentally and to express the full range of one's potentialities. The preamble of the charter of the World Health Organization attempts to convey this utopian ideal in the following words: 'Health is a state of complete physical, mental, and social well-

being and not merely the absence of disease or infirmity.'
Health so defined is a utopian state indeed.

Health will be considered in the following pages from a
more practical point of view, not as an ideal state of well-being
achieved through the complete elimination of disease, but as
a modus vivendi enabling imperfect men to achieve a reward-
ing and not too painful existence while they cope with an imperfect world. In this light, health cannot be defined in the
absolute, because different persons expect such different things
from life. A Wall Street executive, a lumberjack in the Cana-
dian Rockies, a newspaper boy at a crowded street corner, a
steeplechase jockey, a cloistered monk, and the pilot of a
supersonic combat plane have various physical and mental
needs. The imperfections and limitations of the flesh and of
the mind do not have equal importance for them. Their goals
determine the kind of vigour and resistance required for success in their own lives.

A farmer's wife with several children and a New York
fashion model of the same age also differ in their physical requirements and therefore have divergent concepts of health.
The history of fashions and contemporary tastes reveal how
wide is the gamut of men's views on the ideal feminine figure
and complexion in the course of time and how they still differ
from one country to the other. The fleshiness of Paleolithic
'Venuses' or of Rubens' goddesses reflects an attitude toward
womanhood, at least toward female anatomy, oddly different
from the tastes that generated the slender English pre-
Raphaelite models in the nineteenth century or American flap-
pers in the 1920s.

Granted the theoretical impossibility of defining the words
health and disease in a manner acceptable to all, history records a few situations where human beings seem to have
achieved a seemingly healthy state of physical development by
usual criteria. In the account of his travels, Christopher Columbus expressed great admiration for the beautiful physical
state of the Carib Indians he had discovered. Similarly, Captain Cook, Bougainville and the other early explorers of the

Pacific Islands marvelled at the health and physical beauty of the various Polynesian populations.

It is worth noting that human beings with the most nearly ideal state of physical health belonged to rather primitive societies removed from the main channels of human affairs. The Eskimo tribes constitute examples of such isolated groups reputed to have enjoyed glowing health and great vigour despite the harshness of their environment and the primitiveness of their ways of life. In all cases, however, those healthy primitive peoples described in their native habitats by explorers rapidly underwent physical decadence upon contact with the white man and the deleterious influence of his ways of life. Some of the accounts of primitive tribes by explorers and medical anthropologists are well documented; they present a picture of human life so different from the one seen in modern societies that they are of extreme importance for the understanding of the determinants of health and disease. It seems useful, therefore, to review briefly at this point what is known concerning the medical problems of ancient and primitive man.

Health and Disease Among Primitive Peoples

In the course of evolution, as his characteristic structural, physiological and mental equipment gradually emerged, ancient man developed the fitness to resist environmental threats, those dangers emanating from cosmic forces, food shortages, microbial parasites, wild animals or human competitors.

Most of the skeletal remains found in Paleolithic and Neolithic sites are of vigorous adults essentially free of organic diseases at the time of death. Human remains of more recent origin provide further evidence of primitive man's ability to resist harsh natural conditions, at least until he is exposed to influences of Western civilization. A large burial ground from a period preceding Captain Cook's discovery of the Hawaiian Islands was recently excavated in Honolulu; the skeletons recovered from the site had healthy teeth and strong bones with powerful muscle attachments. Apparently life on the Hawaiian Islands was compatible with health and vigour even under the primitive conditions of pre-European settlements. Similar discoveries made in other parts of the world validate the legend of the healthy, happy savage appearing in accounts of primitive life written by seventeenth- and eighteenth-century explorers.

Recent medical surveys of contemporary African, American Indian and Australian tribes give us even more convincing evidence that health and vigour can be achieved under primitive conditions in extremely harsh climates. During the 1960s Western physicians, biologists and anthropologists studied the Meban Negroes of East Africa and the Chavanté Indians of the Brazilian Mato Grosso in their own undisturbed environments. The Meban and Chavanté tribes live in isolated primitive villages, with limited food resources, under difficult climatic conditions and out of contact with Western technology or medicine. Men in both tribes were found to be extremely vigorous and of magnificent physique. They were essentially free from dental caries, high blood pressure, cancer and other degenerative diseases so common in civilized, prosperous countries.

The medical and social picture seen by modern scientists in these two primitive tribes parallels in many respects the description of Eskimo life during the early decades of this century published by various explorers. Modern findings in this regard are also reminiscent of eighteenth-century descriptions by voyagers in Oceania and in the Americas. Granted the likelihood that early explorers and contemporary medical investigators failed to detect many disease problems common among the primitive people they observed or studied, their testimony makes clear nevertheless that health and vigour can be achieved in the absence of modern sanitation and without the help of Western medicine. Man has in his nature the potentiality to reach a high level of physical and mental well-being even without nutritional abundance or physical comfort.

While there is no doubt that man can become adapted to

the dangerous conditions of primitive life, almost nothing is known of the precise mechanisms through which this state of adaptedness is achieved. Furthermore, it must not be assumed from the foregoing rosy picture of primitive health that disease occurs only under the conditions of civilized life and would inevitably disappear if human beings were willing to return to the ways of nature. Many facts militate against this conclusion.

Very few of the prehistoric skeletons discovered so far are of human beings who were old at the time of death. Judged from information available at present, ancient man rarely lived much beyond the age of fifty. The medical study of the Chavanté Indians mentioned above has led to a similar conclusion. Although the men of this tribe are in general vigorous and healthy, seemingly only a small percentage of them reach old age. These concordant findings have been explained away by the hypothesis that death among primitive people comes not from disease or senility but from violent causes such as accidents or homicide. As yet unproven, this hypothesis does not preclude the possibility that pathological processes still unrecognized are responsible for the short life span of many people living under primitive conditions.

Several investigators have recently called attention to the scarcity of cancers, vascular disorders and other degenerative diseases among the most carefully studied primitive populations. Unfortunately, so few old people existed in most of these populations that the significance of such findings is unclear. Since neoplastic, vascular and degenerative disorders become prevalent only in late adulthood, few men and women in primitive populations live long enough to become victims of them. Also, as we shall again emphasize later, the health, vigour and resistance of primitive people is often almost an artifact resulting from the selective processes. The unfit are weeded out, and only those members of the tribe endowed with great innate resistance survive. Life under primitive conditions helps human beings become stronger and tougher, but it is obvious that those who are seen and counted are the favoured ones who have survived precisely because they had the innate attributes to become strong and tough.

Finally, a vigorous and healthy appearance does not necessarily imply the absence of disease. Resistant as they had to be in order to survive, ancient populations nevertheless experienced many of the diseases that afflict mankind today. Skeletons obtained from the Paeolithic sites or Neolithic settlements, the Egyptian mummies, the drawings, sculptures, and other artifacts from the most ancient civilizations in Africa, Asia, Europe and America all provide overwhelming evidence that many of the diseases known today have long existed and probably have been coeval with human life. A list of the medical conditions recognized in the remains of prehistoric and primitive man reads like the catalogue of a pathological museum in a modern medical school.

It is almost impossible to establish with certainty whether mental diseases existed among the most ancient people, but descriptions of abnormal behaviour and illustrations of hysteria in early Greek literature and art leave no doubt that disorders of the mind have long been accompaniments of human life. Many forms of mental disease are frequent also among primitive populations today.

The problem of health and disease among primitive peoples thus presents itself under two different aspects. Prehistoric remains and ancient history strongly suggest that disease has been coexistent with human life; other kinds of anthropological evidence indicate that life under the most primitive conditions is compatible with a high level of health. This incompatibility of evidence is more apparent than real. Disease can occur occasionally in one person without affecting his group as a whole. Recognition of a particular disease in a Paleolithic or Neolithic skeleton does not signify its prevalence in prehistoric communities.

Equally important, the achievement of a healthy state depends in large part upon man's ability to become well adapted to a stable environment. At the time of their discovery by white men, the societies of Polynesians, American Indians,

Eskimos and other primitive peoples were in a state of arrested civilization. For long periods of time they had lived in fairly stable physical and social environments almost out of contact with the rest of mankind. They had achieved an equilibrium with their limited world and learned to utilize its natural food resources and to protect themselves against its threats. In particular, they had developed a high level of immunity against the microbial agents of disease prevalent in their communities.

Adaptive fitness similarly accounts for the health of wild animals in their natural habitats. Both men and animals achieve health most readily after many generations of life in a stable environment; health persists only as long as conditions remain undisturbed. The healthy savages described by the explorers belonged to tribes living in isolation at the time of their discovery, tribes well adapted to their native and unchanging physical and social environment.

Social Upheavals and Disease Causation

From historical experience, we know that all primitive peoples fall prey to many forms of disease when they come into contact with Western civilization. The details of this increased susceptibility to disease are complex, but the general pattern is quite simple.

Whenever European explorers entered a newly discovered country, they unwittingly introduced a host of microbes they harboured in their bodies. These microbes, little harming the Europeans who had built up resistance to them, proved highly virulent for the primitive peoples who had had no prior contact with them. Not only did the Europeans introduce new infectious agents but their arrival and continued presence suddenly and profoundly disturbed the nutritional habits and ancestral ways of life of the primitive tribes. These social disturbances further lowered general resistance to disease. Such a constellation of unfavourable circumstances readily accounts for the immensely destructive character of the diseases that afflicted the Polynesians, the American Indians and the Eskimos during the eighteenth, nineteenth and twentieth centuries. (Parenthetically, the reverse process is also true. That is, many Europeans who go to primitive areas commonly encounter infectious agents to which they have no acquired resistance and to which they fall prey. It is thought, though not proven, that syphilis came to Europe by this process following the New World explorations of Columbus.)

In Europe and America, all periods of social upheaval have been accompanied by a marked increase in the incidence of disease and, more strikingly, by a change in the relative incidence of various kinds of diseases. During the nineteenth century the circumstances surrounding the Industrial Revolution brought on an explosive aggravation of many pathological states with a resulting deterioration of general health, especially among the labouring classes. Within a few decades, millions of men and women migrated from rural districts into mushrooming industrial cities where they had to live under physiologically deplorable and totally strange conditions. We shall later mention specific factors acting as direct causes of disease; it will suffice here to emphasize that the industrial environment per se constituted the primary disturbing factor. Because it was unhealthy and different from anything experienced before, it imposed on the immigrants recently arrived from rural areas, especially from foreign countries, excessive adaptive demands that they could not meet successfully.

Whatever their nationality, the citizens of prosperous countries have by now become fairly well adapted to the kinds of environment emergent from the first Industrial Revolution. This does not mean, however, that failures of adaptations are no longer important in the causation of disease among Westernized people. Environmental conditions change constantly and rapidly, partly because we manipulate them in an attempt to control the external world and more perhaps because each technological and social innovation has unpredictable consequences. These unforeseen effects alter many aspects of our lives, often in an unfavourable manner. The more dynamic the society, the more rapid and profound are the modifications in environment and ways of life. As many persons fail to meet successfully the adaptive requirements created by these rapidly changing conditions, numerous and varied pathological states emerge despite an increase in comfort and prosperity.

The experience of modern life shows that most social or technological changes engender either immediate or delayed physiological disturbances and can act as direct or indirect causes of disease. Before proceeding further with this theme, however, it seems necessary to define the word *cause* with greater care, because, as we shall presently see, its meaning is far more complex than commonly assumed.

Theories of Disease Causation

The reader consulting an encyclopedia about the cause of a particular disease is likely to receive an equivocal answer. And surprising as it may seem, he may not obtain more definite information from professional textbooks of medicine, for, in most cases, there is no simple answer. Much is known of the anatomical and functional abnormalities behind the signs and symptoms of disease, but information is often lacking on the causative circumstances initially associated with these changes. The common cold illustrates how conceptual difficulties with the very meaning of the word 'cause' can compound the scientific task of identifying specific causation.

As its name indicates, the common cold is a very 'common' disease. Consequently, almost every person has opinions on the circumstances that bring it about. The 'cold' is so called since, in experience, it is more likely to develop during periods of bad weather, especially when the temperature suddenly falls. The discovery a few decades ago that groups of men isolated for several months in Arctic posts usually remained free of the common cold until the arrival of a ship made it clear that the common cold is not necessarily associated with bad weather. Confirmed time and time again, this observation has made it clear that low temperatures or inclement weather cannot alone produce the common cold; a more likely hypothesis is that the illness follows infection by a microbe. This hypothesis is of course compatible with general experience, since almost everyone believes that a cold is 'catching'.

Recent experiments, designed to show that a condition similar to the common cold can be produced by spraying suspensions of certain viruses into the nostrils of human volunteers, have substantiated the microbial theory of cold causation. According to present evidence, numerous strains of virus can cause these symptoms, a finding obviously and disturbingly pointing to the existence of a multiplicity of microbial causative agents. To complicate the microbial theory further, many volunteers fail to develop a cold even though they have been heavily contaminated with virus suspensions known to cause the disease in other persons. Other experiments have revealed still more complexities. The chance of contracting a cold is not appreciably increased when volunteers wearing wet socks in a drafty, cold room, conditions assumed by both physicians and laymen to enhance susceptibility, are exposed to the implicated viruses.

Exposure to one of several viruses is a *necessary* condition for the development of the common cold but not a *sufficient* condition. Exposure results in disease only when the exposed person is in a receptive state. This receptivity is in turn affected by the season, the weather, and almost certainly by a host of other ill-defined factors, such as fatigue, probably acting to decrease general resistance to infection.

The puzzle of the common cold, and of its multifactorial determinants, has its counterpart in most important diseases. Indeed, multifactorial etiology is the rule rather than the exception, and apparently conflicting theories of disease causation can be reconciled. Several decades ago, scientists discovered that cancers can be produced by exposure to certain substances such as tar and a host of synthetic products called carcinogenic for precisely this reason. Many recent experiments have proven, on the other hand, that cancer can also be produced in animals by exposing them to radium or X rays, by injecting them with an ovarian hormone and by infecting them with certain viruses. Finally, it has been shown that hereditary factors, hormonal secretions, and various other physiological agencies can influence the development of cancer following exposure to carcinogenic substances or to viruses. Judging from past experience, it can be safely predicted that the present piecemeal succession of apparently conflicting statements on the cause of neoplastic diseases will eventually be replaced by the larger view that several factors, acting simultaneously, are usually instrumental in their causation.

Multifactorial etiology is involved also in vascular disorders. Excess of saturated fats and of cholesterol in the diet, lack of physical exercise, the tensions of modern life, and hereditary factors all play a part in the rising incidence of heart disease in prosperous communities. In this case again, it will probably be found that constitutional factors and several different aspects of the ways of life, including food intake and energy expenditure, play a part in altering the structure of the blood vessels and in determining at critical times the size of the load that they can handle with safety.

In almost all cases, several determinant factors must therefore act in concert to produce a detectable pathological state; moreover, the manifestations of any given agent differ profoundly from one person to another. Thus, causality and specificity are much less readily demonstrated in natural clinical situations than they are in experimental laboratory models. Admittedly, a few acute infectious processes and nutritional deficiencies present such a characteristic clinical picture that there is no difficulty in identifying them and in attributing them to specific causes. Few diseases present such a simple picture. What the patient experiences and what the physician observes constitute generally a confusing variety of symptoms and lesions rather than a well-defined entity. In most cases, a complex syndrome such as anaemia, cardiac insufficiency, gastric disturbance or depression is more in evidence than the unique and clear-cut pathological manifestations of a specific etiological agent.

In common experience, a traumatic accident that would be fatal to an aged person may have only trivial consequences for a young healthy adult. More generally, the character and severity of the damage caused by any given deleterious agency will differ from one situation to another. The pulmonary disease that our nineteenth-century ancestors called a decline, consumption or phthisis was unquestionably pulmonary tuberculosis; but it was usually much more severe than the kind of tuberculosis most commonly seen in our communities today. Evidence indicates that the virulence of tubercle bacilli has not changed; what has changed is the response of Western man to tuberculous infection. Many other examples could be quoted to illustrate that the severity of a microbial or toxic disease is determined as much by the intensity of the body response as it is by the characteristics of the microbe or toxin involved.

Noxious agents differing widely in nature can elicit similar reactions from the body, complicating still further an understanding of disease causation. Congestion of the nasal mucous membranes and their hypersecretion can be caused by many unrelated agencies such as viral and bacterial infections; inhalation of smoke, dust, allergens or cold air; migraine of vascular origin; the administration of certain drugs; sorrow and tears. Likewise, urticaria can result from contact with wool, from consumption of many types of foods and drugs, from emotional disturbances, or from exposure to agents as different as sunlight and cold. Bacterial endocarditis in man and mastitis in cows used to be caused almost exclusively by streptococci. Now that streptococcal infections can be successfully treated with penicillin, other microbial species commonly establish themselves in the heart lesions of human beings or in the mammary lesions of cows; they thus give a new microbial causation to these ancient diseases.

The body is capable of only a limited range of reactions. Its response to assaults of very different origin and nature is consequently rather stereotyped. Intestinal lesions mimicking those of typhoid fever can be produced by introducing into the mesenteric nodes of animals almost any irritating substance, even a rose thorn. Stimulation of the neurovegetative system can produce severe lesions not only in the viscera directly affected but also in others with indirect and distant anatomical connexions. So much uniformity in the lesions and hormonal responses caused by various types of noxious stimuli has been observed that the blanket expressions 'stress response' and, more technically, 'General Adaptation Syndrome' have been coined to include them all. Such uniformity of response seems incompatible with the doctrine of specific causation. Were it only for this reason, there is need for a new formulation of the etiological theory.

The activities of various hormones influence all of the human organism's responses to noxious agencies. The secretion of these hormones is in turn affected by psychological factors and by the symbolic interpretation the mind attaches to environmental agents and stimuli. This individual interpretation is so profoundly conditioned by the experiences of the past and by the anticipations of the future that the physicochemical characteristics of noxious agents rarely determine the character of the pathological processes they set in motion. These facts also point to the need and the possibility of reformulating theories of disease causation.

In its original form the doctrine of specificity was focused on a few external agents of disease, such as microbes, poisons, traumatic accidents, nutritional deficiences and ionizing radiations. In the light of modern findings, etiological theories must concern themselves not only with the direct effects of noxious factors on the target organs but also with the factors such as hormonal actions or mental processes governing the responses of the human organism.

The response to any noxious influence usually involves the organism as a whole, and, as a result, it is rarely possible to account for the natural processes of disease in terms of simple and direct cause-effect relationships. The external environment and the *milieu intérieur* constitute a multifactorial system, each component of which must be studied for its own characteristics and for its effects on the other components of the system. The concept of multifactorial causation does not discredit the classical doctrine of specificity. Rather, it constitutes an extension of it and brings scientific understanding a little nearer to the complexities of the real world.

Like living organisms, theories can survive only by adapting themselves to new demands and by continuously evolving. If the doctrine of causality were restricted to its classical formulation, it would wither away or at best become mummified. Thomas Huxley, in his statement that new truths commonly begin as heresies but all too often end as superstitions, pungently expressed this danger a century ago. Fortunately, the doctrine of specific etiology is acquiring new life and becoming even more fruitful of understanding because its scope is being widened. At first focused on a few noxious factors of the external world, it is now taking cognizance of a multiplicity of internal mechanisms when body and mind attempt to respond adaptively to environmental stimuli and stresses. Failure of such adaptive efforts accounts for a large percentage of diseases. Seen from this broader point of view, the doctrine of specificity will stimulate the development of methods for the study of the whole human organism's response to the presence of any noxious agent. It will thus permit a more comprehensive analysis of the multifarious mechanisms involved in disease causation. 'Science,' Pasteur wrote, 'advances through tentative answers to a series of more and more subtle questions which reach deeper and deeper into the essence of natural phenomena.'

Changing Patterns of Disease

As we have seen, diseases most prevalent in modern industrialized nations also afflicted prehistoric man and exist today in all primitive societies; diseases have unchangeable and universal characters because man's nature has remained essentially the same for some one hundred thousand years. The relative prevalence of the various diseases, however, has changed from one historical period to another and differs today among geographical areas and social groups. Differences in the total environment and in the ways of life make for this diversity.

Many kinds of documents testify to spectacular change in the prevalence and severity of diseases during historical times. The classical texts from India, Greece or Rome contain numerous and accurate descriptions of the signs and symptoms of advanced pulmonary tuberculosis, a disease almost rampant in ancient urban civilizations. In contrast, neither the Old nor the New Testament contains references to tuberculosis, probably because these texts constitute the lore of pastoral peoples whose ways of life made them resistant to this disease. Countless paintings and drawings illustrating the manifestations and ravages of plague document the frequent occurrence of this disease in Europe from the fourteenth to the seventeenth century. Boccaccio's *Decameron* and Daniel Defoe's *A Journal of the Plague Year* underscore the severity of bubonic plague during that period in Europe. Plague practically disappeared thereafter from Europe, though it is still today a destructive scourge in many parts of Asia.

Rowlandson, Gillray, Daumier and many other nineteenth-century artists have documented in their caricatures the frequency of gout and of gross obesity among the prosperous and overfed bourgeois of their times in England and in France. Novelists and social reformers of the same period have left us dramatic acounts of the appalling physiologic misery among the labouring classes in Western Europe during the early phases of the Industrial Revolution. In *The Condition of the Working Class in England*, Engels wrote of the 'pale, lank, narrow-chested, hollow-eyed ghosts', riddled with scrofula and rickets, who haunted the streets of Manchester and other manufacturing towns.

If ever man lived under conditions completely removed from the state of nature dreamed of by Rousseau and his followers, it was English proletariat of the 1830s. Public-minded citizens came to believe that, since disease always accompanied want, dirt and pollution, the best and perhaps the only way to improve health was to bring back to the multitudes pure air, pure water, pure food and pleasant surroundings. As we shall see later, this point of view relates directly to the problems of disease being created in the modern world by the second Industrial Revolution, and to their control by social improvements.

In nineteenth-century Europe, the sanitary ideal developed at first without any support from laboratory science. It emerged from the conviction that with the correction of filth, dirt, crowding and other social ills, high rates of disease and death could be prevented also. Simple as was this concept, it would not have become a creative force in medicine and in public health if it had not been publicized and implemented by intensely dedicated social reformers. Their crusade brought about a true sanitary revolution resulting unquestionably in the practical control of many diseases, especially those affecting the multitudes. Nothing demonstrates more vividly the profound changes that can occur within a few generations in the health of a people. One has only to contrast the sickly proletariat described by Engels and the tall, husky men now typical of the working classes in prosperous Western countries to appreciate what miracles can be wrought in a short time.

The pages of history do not provide the only evidence of disease patterns differing and changing rapidly with environmental and social conditions. A most spectacular proof of this relationship emerges from a comparison of mortality and morbidity rates, as well as of types of diseases, recorded in our own times for different countries and different social groups. Today as in the past, each civilization has its own characteristic pattern of diseases determined by its climate, its customs, its technology and its living standards.

Disease presents itself simultaneously with so many different faces in any given area that it is usually impossible to attribute one particular expression of it to one particular set of environmental circumstances. Nevertheless, some generalizations appear justified. Without question, nutritional and infectious diseases account for the largest percentage of morbidity and mortality in most underprivileged countries, especially in those just becoming industrialized. Undernutrition, protein deficiency, malaria, tuberculosis, infestation with worms, and a host of ill-defined gastrointestinal disorders are today the greatest killers in these countries, just as they used to be in the Western world one century ago. In contrast, the toll taken by malnutrition and infection decreases rapidly wherever and whenever the living standards improve, but other diseases then become more prevalent. In prosperous countries at the present time, heart diseases constitute the leading cause of death, with cancers in the second place, vascular lesions affecting the central nervous system in the third, and accidents in the fourth. Increasingly also, persons who are well fed and well sheltered suffer from a variety of chronic disorders, such as arthritis and allergies, that do not destroy life but often ruin it.

Disease as Affected by the Ways of Life

We now have sufficient knowledge to provide fairly rational explanations for the changes that have occurred and continue to occur in the patterns of disease. Mechanistic explanations are rarely sufficient to account for pathological phenomena unless they take into consideration the role of social and ethical factors. A few examples taken from the past and from recent history may help to illustrate the intimate relationships that exist between the nature of man, his beliefs, his behaviour and his diseases.

Epidemics and other disease manifestations have been interpreted since ancient times as punishment for collective or individual sin. The well-documented cases of death by suggestion in primitive tribes when a man broke a taboo or some other tribal regulation can be traced to this ancient belief. In all probability, voodoo death is but an extreme form of body response to fear or panic and has its counterpart in even the most advanced communities. In the minds of many persons everywhere disease is still associated with guilt.

The outbreak of Manchurian plague at the turn of this century constitutes a well-documented example of the role of living patterns in disease causation. The plague bacillus is widely distributed among the wild rodents of Asia. Manchurian marmots normally harbour this microbe, but they do not suffer from the infection under usual circumstances. Around 1910, a change in women's fashions in Europe suddenly created a large demand for the fur of the Manchurian marmot, and a number of inexperienced Chinese hunters began to hunt this wild rodent. Until then it had been hunted only by Manchurians who had a taboo forbidding them to hunt sick animals. In contrast, the inexperienced Chinese trapped every animal within reach, especially the sickest who were slower and easier to catch. As it turned out, the sick marmots were suffering from plague, and many Chinese hunters contracted the infection from them. When the hunters met in the crowded and ill-ventilated Manchurian inns, those who had caught the microbe spread it to their neighbours, thereby initiating a widespread epidemic of pneumonic plague. A change in women's fashions in Europe thus indirectly caused an epidemic of pneumonic plague in Manchuria.

It might be thought that women's fashions, Manchurian marmots, crowded inns and pneumonic plague constitute such an artificial and unusual concatenation of circumstances that nothing comparable could possibly occur in highly organized and sophisticated societies. Overwhelming evidence indicates quite the contrary; many forms of disease have emerged or have been disseminated in the modern world because our ways of life have created new and complex constellations of circumstances favourable for their spread.

Porphyria, an affliction which damages the red blood cells, illustrates how modern innovations can result in new forms of disease. This hereditary disorder originated with a Dutch woman who migrated to South Africa in 1686. As far as is known, the gene for porphyria has been transmitted ever since to all her descendants; although these are now numerous, the disease itself has become a problem only during recent years. Under ordinary conditions, the porphyria gene manifests itself only by the production of mild neurological symptoms and minor skin blemishes usually overlooked. However, violent reactions often culminating in death are likely to occur if the porphyric person takes certain modern drugs such as sulfas and barbiturates. The normally mild signs and symptoms of this genetic disorder are converted suddenly into severe and often fatal responses by modern drugs otherwise considered lifesaving.

Porphyria is an extreme case of a general biomedical phenomenon. Most genetic abnormalities result in severe disease only under certain environmental conditions. Susceptibility to diabetes is genetically inherited. The manifestations of the disease are usually severe among persons whose diet is rich and abundant. During the Second World War diabetes became much milder among the Europeans in concentration camps or in other areas where the supply of food was limited. Analogous situations relating environment to disease could probably be worked out for almost any genetic disorder.

Some geneticists have even postulated that obesity, correlated in our prosperous communities with great susceptibility to disease and a short life expectancy, may have constituted a genetic advantage in the distant past when the supply of food was erratic and when man often had to depend on his bodily reserves for survival. This hypothesis finds no convincing evidence, but its merit is to illustrate that in all cases the deleterious manifestations of a gene are profoundly conditioned by environmental influences.

The Diseases of Civilization

Cancer, heart disease and disorders of the cerebral system are commonly referred to as diseases of civilization. Strictly speaking, the designation is incorrect, since these diseases occur also among the primitive peoples but such chronic and degenerative conditions are so much more frequent among prosperous peoples than among primitive or economically deprived groups that it is justifiable to speak of 'diseases of civilization'. The very use of the phrase is tacit acknowledgement that our ways of life may have nefarious effects and that affluence, like poverty, can constitute a cause of disease.

Experiments with animals and observation of human beings have established beyond doubt that cancer can be produced by agencies as different as viruses, ionizing radiations, tar products and a multiplicity of unrelated chemical substances. The precise mechanisms through which these agencies bring about uncontrolled neoplastic growths are still obscure. Granted this uncertainty, the conclusion is inescapable: many types of neoplastic disease can be traced to several different kinds of environmental factors. While all human beings can develop cancers, the incidence of various types of this disease exhibits spectacular differences from one country and one social group to another. Lung cancer is the most common cause of cancer death among men in the United States, England, Wales and several other Western countries, but it is much less frequent in Iceland. In contrast, stomach cancer accounts for 50 per cent of cancers among men in Iceland and Japan but for only 10 per cent in the United States and for even less in Indonesia. Liver cancer causes half of all cancer deaths among the Bantus in Africa but less than 4 per cent in Europe and North America. Breast cancer is over eight times more common among women in Israel than among women in Japan. Cancer of the cervix accounts for half of all cancer deaths among Hindu women.

Local differences also exist within a given country. Skin and lip cancers are proportionately twenty times more common among white people living in the southern half of the United States than among those living in the northern half. In the U.S.S.R., they are five to six times more common in the south than in the north and are particularly frequent on the coast itself. One is reminded here of Hemingway's character in *The Old Man and the Sea* with his precancerous lesions on the face. These peculiarities in cancer distribution cannot be explained in terms of the race or colour of the peoples involved. All evidence points rather to the ways of life as the responsible agents – perhaps simply extensive exposure to sunshine. The rapid increase in the incidence of lung carcinoma in our communities and the concomitant decrease in the incidence of stomach cancer leave no doubt that, while all human beings are potentially susceptible to neoplastic disease, environmental factors primarily determine its frequency and manifestations.

A similar conclusion can be reached from the study of the prevalence of vascular diseases. Enormous geographical and social differences exist in the distribution of deaths caused by vascular disorders, but it is now certain that racial factors are not involved. Differences in frequency are at least as great among the various economic strata of a given race in a given country as they are among national groups. Vascular diseases are rare among Chinese coolies, among the Navaho Indians who have remained on their reservations, and among Negroes still living in primitive African villages. In contrast, they are common among the Chinese, Navahos and Negroes who have adopted the ways of life of prosperous industrialized and urbanized people.

Nutritional excesses, lack of physical exercise, emotional tension, excessive smoking and other deleterious habits can have disastrous consequences in persons with abnormal lipid and cholesterol metabolism and can thereby elicit vascular disease. Admittedly, little is known concerning the physiological mechanisms of these interrelationships, but the point of importance here is that the occurrence of vascular disease, like that of cancer, is conditioned by many factors of the total environment.

The ways of life also play a part in the causation of mental diseases. Comparative studies of different parts of the world and of different economic groups show the propensity to behavioural disturbances to be more or less uniform among all races. Here again the frequency of these disturbances is socially conditioned. Anguish or social pressures, according to the evidence, can provoke overt mental disease in persons having slight abnormalities of the nervous system, aberrations compatible with socially acceptable behaviour under more favourable emotional or social circumstances.

Whereas micorbiological pollution of water used to be responsible for much disease among our ancestors, chemical pollution of the air is now becoming a great public health problem. Chemical fumes from factories and motor vehicle exhausts are causing a variety of pathological disorders that threaten to increase in frequency and gravity. They may create widespread and serious health handicaps in the near future. There is reason to fear that various types of ionizing radiation will soon add their long-range and unpredictable effects to this pathology of the future.

During recent decades we have gone far toward controlling microbial spoilage of food, but some of the new synthetic products ubiquitous in modern life are responsible for an endless variety of allergic and toxic effects.

Nutritional deficiencies are now a rarity in the prosperous countries of the world, but a new kind of malnutrition is rising. Nutritional regimens formulated for physically active human beings are no longer suited to automobile-borne, air-conditioned and automated life in the twentieth century.

In the past many human beings suffered from physical exhaustion; now labour-saving devices and dial-controlled operations threaten to generate types of psychiatric disturbances likely to complicate the medicine of tomorrow. Boredom is replacing fatigue.

Who could have dreamed a generation ago that hypervitaminoses (conditions arising from an excess of certain vitamins) would become a nutritional disease in the Western world; that the introduction of detergents and various other synthetics would increase the incidence of allergies; that advances in chemotherapy and other therapeutic procedures would create new forms of microbial disease; that patients suffering from toxicities induced by drugs would occupy such a large number of beds in modern hospitals; that cigarettes, air pollutants and ionizing radiations would be held responsible for the increase in certain types of cancer; that some maladies of our times could be referred to as 'pathology of inactivity' and 'occupational hazards of sedentary and light work'?

It can be taken for granted that, while man's nature will remain fundamentally the same as it has been since Paleolithic times, the pattern of his diseases will continue to change because his physiological responses to changing environmental situations will not adapt him rapidly enough to the new conditions. Change itself may constitute a cause of disease. Once man is adapted to certain kinds of food, weather, housing, microbes and social habits, he commonly finds it unpleasant and traumatic to be uprooted suddenly and forced to live under new conditions even though these appear more favourable to the outsider. As Hippocrates wrote two and a half thousand years ago, 'It is changes that are chiefly responsible for diseases, especially the greatest changes, the violent alterations both in the seasons and in other things.'

Mechanisms of Adaptation

The physiological characteristics of man strongly indicate that his early evolution took place in a subtropical environment, probably at low altitudes. In the absence of clothing, housing, shelter or other means of protection, human beings usually feel most comfortable at a temperature approximating 29° C (about 85°F), with moderate humidity and little air movement. In general, men make physiological adjustments much more readily to tropical than to Arctic conditions; adjustments to life in cold climates depend on the use of technological and social devices rather than on true biological adaptation.

Man began to migrate extensively and to colonize most of the globe during the Late Paleolithic period. As he dispersed away from the conditions of his biological origins, he underwent many deep-seated anatomical and physiological adaptative changes, and the progressive emergence of the several human races took place. Migrations on a large scale, and successful settlement in remote areas, became possible only after man had mastered certain technologies and social procedures permitting him to survive and to function effectively under profoundly altered climatic conditions. The success of man as a species is a consequence of his ability to call into play a wide range of adaptive potentialities.

For man, as for other living things, the word 'adaptation' connotes fitness to a particular environment or the possession of attributes making it possible to function effectively and to reproduce abundantly in this environment. Adaptation, however, is often bought at a high price, and its consequences may be unfavourable in the long run. Therein lies the reason for one of the most paradoxical aspects of human life. On the one hand, it is certain that the diversity and immensity of man's achievements stem in large part from his lack of biological specialization and his gift for adaptation, the greatest among mammals. On the other hand, these same attributes create many of his biological and social difficulties.

Animals in the wild achieve adaptation to their environment chiefly through genetic mechanisms. This was certainly the case also for the early precursors of man, probably until they reached the level of *Homo sapiens*. For a long time after his emergence, early man also had to depend on the attributes of his genetic endowment to overcome the countless dangers to which he was constantly exposed. Early death of the unfit or their failure to leave a progeny assured the selective reproduction of human types endowed with the attributes best fitted to the various environments in which men settled during the prehistoric period. Selective environmental influences moulded innate differences in body shape, in skin pigmentation, and even in emotional temperament. Gradually, as men migrated to different regions, they divided into biologically and socially separate groups.

In the course of time, and probably even before he had

completed his biological evolution, man learned to function in complex social groups and to use fire, tools, clothing and shelter. He was thus able to supplement his genetic mechanisms with social procedures. Naturally, he long remained threatened by certain dangers, especially those resulting from infection and shortages of food. Wherever the environment is harsh, the food resources limited and the ways of life unsanitary, a large percentage of the population dies during infancy, childhood and early adulthood. Under such conditions, today as in the past, the constant weeding out of those most susceptible to malnutrition and to infection naturally brings about selective breeding for a high degree of native resistance to certain forms of infectious and nutritional disease.

Genetic mechanisms of resistance to disease have their drawbacks, however. Natural resistance acquired through genetic selection is effective chiefly, if not entirely, for the conditions under which it is selected; it is of little value in another environment or when the ways of life change. Genetic resistance to one type of disease may entail greater susceptibility to another. In many parts of Africa and around the Mediterranean, certain genetic peculiarities affecting the composition of the blood pigment haemoglobin are associated with greater resistance to malaria and therefore are advantageous wherever this disease is endemic. What is an asset where malaria is endemic, however, becomes a handicap in the United States where it has been almost eradicated. The defect in haemoglobin mentioned above may express itself in the form of a serious disease, sickle-cell anaemia.

An even greater drawback of genetic resistance achieved through the weeding out by death of the least fit persons is that it is very costly in human lives. Fortunately, genetic adaptation can be supplemented by other biological mechanisms not involving sacrifice of human life and more rapid in their effects. Tanning increases resistance to solar radiation; immunity acquired through early exposure or through vaccination minimizes the effects of infectious agents and certain poisons; continued life at high altitude results in greater ability to live and work in an atmosphere deficient in oxygen; controlled exercise in humid heat improves the ability to function under tropical conditions; practice develops most physical attributes and skills as well as the ability to learn or to endure pain. The mechanisms of such physiological adaptations do not entail a modification of the genetic endowment; yet the physiological and behavioural characteristics acquired by individuals through experience during life are an essential part of adaptation.

While genetic and physiological mechanisms of adaptation continue to operate in man, the control of the environment through technology progressively decreases their importance and in some cases appears to make them obsolete. Control of water and food supplies, better ventilation of dwellings and various procedures of sanitation have greatly reduced the spread of many killing infectious agents and have almost eliminated the role of infection as a selective force in human evolution. Poor eyesight is less and less a biological handicap because it can be corrected by glasses. Insulin enables diabetics to live as long as other persons and to have as many children. Even phenylketonuria, a genetic disease resulting a few years ago in death or gross mental disability, can now be partially controlled by proper dietary management. Modern man can so manipulate his environment and the conditions of his life to minimize the effects of genetic abnormalities and postpone death from the diseases they cause. Needless to say, such manipulations interfere with or prevent altogether the operation of natural selective processes.

Environmental control also decreases the need for physiological adaptations. Man finds it more convenient to air-condition his dwellings than to adapt physiologically to heat or cold; wherever possible, he uses mechanical devices instead of depending on his muscles; he invents learning aids to decrease mental effort; he takes drugs as a substitute for mental discipline in resisting pain and overcoming fatigue. Almost universally, man tries to eliminate the unpleasant effects of environmental forces instead of making the greater effort required to cope with them through his own adaptive physiological resources.

Man's control of the environment has gone further than his biological adaptabilities toward eliminating many forms of suffering; it has thus constituted one of the most influential determinants of civilization. Yet it is a dangerous error to believe that disease and suffering can be wiped out altogether by raising still further the standards of living, increasing our mastery of the environment, and developing new therapeutic procedures. The less pleasant reality is that, since the world is ever changing, each period and each type of civilization will continue to have its burden of diseases created by the unavoidable failure of biological and social adaptation to counter new environmental threats.

The Dangers of Adaptation

Short of nuclear warfare, mankind should be able to take the stresses of the future in its stride just as it has survived destructive famines and epidemics in the past. One can almost take it for granted that mankind will adapt to the new ways of life created by the second Industrial Revolution, and even to the crowding, environmental pollution, shortages of natural resources, and other ordeals likely to result from the rapid increase in the world population.

The potential ability of mankind to survive the threats arising from new technologies and new ways of life constitutes but a limited aspect of the problem of adaptation. Many seemingly fully adaptive biological and social changes desirable today will have to be paid for in the future at a cruel price in terms of human values. A threatening consequence of medical and technological progress is the accumulation in our communities of hereditary defectives, people who today survive into reproductive age and in the past would have died without progeny. Modern ways of life are thus interfering with natural elimination of undesirable genes and are probably creating some measure of genetic hazard. Eventually this widespread impairment of genetic quality will express itself in overt disease or at least in reduced vitality.

It is misleading to speak of biological defectives without regard to the kind of environment in which man lives and functions. While human beings physically handicapped by genetic defects could not long survive under the 'natural' conditions of primitive life, medical and other social techniques enable a biologically 'defective' person to live long and to function effectively in the modern world. Tuberculars, diabetics, blind men, cripples, psychopaths, and those loaded with genes that would be lethal in the wilderness can find useful places in civilized society. Fitness is not an absolute characteristic; it must be defined in terms of the total environment in which the person has to spend his life.

Unfortunately, fitness achieved through constant medical care has distressing social and economic implications for the future. Medicine will certainly continue to progress, but at the same time the cost of medical care will continue to soar. Each new discovery tends to increase the demand for specialized skills and for expensive equipment and products. There is certainly some limit to the percentage of technical and financial resources that society can or will devote to the prevention and treatment of disease.

Technological advances can also exert deleterious nongenetic effects at first unnoticed. Environmental pollution illustrates how many of the adjustments that facilitate life in a hostile environment commonly express themselves later in disease and human misery. The inhabitants of the industrial areas of northern Europe behave as if they had made a successful adjustment to massive air pollution. For more than a century they have functioned effectively and successfully despite irritating substances in the atmosphere they breathe. However, their adaptation is less satisfactory than might be supposed. The lining of their respiratory tracts registers the insult of air pollution. The cumulative effects of years of constant exposure to various pollutants have resulted in widespread chronic bronchitis and other forms of irreversible respiratory disease.

Chronic respiratory disease is now the leading cause of disability among adults in all the industrialized parts of northern Europe and is becoming increasingly prevalent in the United States. This condition provides a model for the kind of medical problems likely to arise in the future from all forms of environmental pollution in industrial communities. Paradoxically, control over the quality of air, water and food is in many cases sufficiently strict to prevent the most obvious kinds of toxic effects. Neither the acute toxicity nor the nuisance value of environmental pollution are great enough to be immediately disabling and to interfere seriously with social and economic life. Public attention is not alerted to the hidden danger of repeated exposure to levels of toxic and irritating agents so low as to remain unnoticed. Like chronic bronchitis, cancer, and many other types of pathological manifestations, the multifarious effects of environmental pollutants may not be detected until several decades after the intial exposure. Many technological innovations certainly exert a variety of unfavourable effects that long remain unnoticed because they are delayed and indirect.

As in the case of environmental pollution, apparently successful adjustments to emotional stresses caused by competitive behaviour and crowding can result in delayed organic and mental disease or at least in behavioural disturbances. Through the experience of social intercourse, man learns to control the outward manifestations of his emotional responses. He usually manages to conceal his impatience, irritations and hostile feelings behind a mask of civil behaviour. Inwardly, however, he still responds to emotional stimuli by means of physiological mechanisms inherited from his Paleolithic ancestry and from his animal past. The ancient fight and flight response still operates in him, calling into play through the autonomic nervous system various hormonal mechanisms that generate useless and potentially dangerous physiological reactions.

The most disturbing aspect of the problem of adaptation is paradoxically that human beings *are* so adaptable. They can become adjusted to conditions and habits that will eventually destroy the values most characteristic of human life. If only for this reason, it is dangerous to apply to human beings the concept of adaptability in a purely biological sense. Biological adaptability often leads to the passive acceptance of conditions in the long run undesirable; the lowest common denominators of existence tend to become the accepted criteria in social and individual life merely for the sake of a grey and anonymous state of peace or tranquillity. There is real danger that the ideal environment will come to be regarded as one in which man is physically comfortable while he progressively forgets the values that constitute the most precious and unique qualities of human life.

In the final analysis, not physical fitness to environmental conditions nor comfort of the body, nor even survival of the human species, suffice to encompass the richness of man's nature. Herein lies the inadequacy of the purely biological view of adaptation. One of the unique characteristics of man is that he does not live only in the present; at his best, he has a deep sense of continuity with the past and is concerned with the future. To be relevant to the human condition, the concept of adaptability must incorporate the needs of day-to-day existence subject to limitations and requirements created by the desire to preserve the past and modified by anticipations for the future.

Medical problems posed by the environmental stimuli and insults of modern civilization have acquired a critical urgency; most technological and social changes now achieve their full effects in a very short time and affect simultaneously almost all parts of the world and all economic classes. Until recently the rate of change was generally so slow as to allow time to make the proper conscious or unconscious adjustments. Many individuals suffered when conditions changed for the worse, but the bulk of mankind slowly and almost unconsciously adapted. The genetic endowment of the population became progressively altered; phenotypic modifications helped each person to function in his particular niche; and, especially, most human beings slowly learned to achieve better fitness to their milieu through technological and social innovations without entirely sacrificing the past or jeopardizing the future. Now the rate of change is so rapid that there may not be time for the orderly and successful operation of these conscious and unconscious adaptive processes. For the first time in the history of mankind, the biological and social experience of the father is almost useless to his son.

5 The Biomedical Control of Human Life

Individual and Collective Aspects of Medical Services

Today the word 'Hospital' suggests an establishment where sick or wounded persons can receive elaborate medical or surgical care. The word has not always had this meaning; it has progessively changed in the course of history; and it will probably continue to change with medical philosophies in the future. The evolving hospital concept provides a striking illustration of changes in public attitude toward disease and in the interplay between individual and collective medicine.

Originally the Latin word *hospitium* referred not to an institution concerned with disease but to a place where a guest was received. The *hospitalia* of the early Middle Ages were essentially guest houses for pilgrims. More and more, hospitals became places where poor people were housed when they were sick or injured. People came to the hospital not so much to be treated as to be protected and decently sheltered.

Institutions of mercy in medieval times were motivated less by the hope of preventing or curing disease through medical intervention than by an attitude of brotherly love in God. This attitude was consonant with the view prevailing during the Middle Ages that disease was primarily a departure from holiness and from spiritual health. In the mind of the medieval scholar and physician there was no dichotomy between mind and body. They treated both physical and mental illness in much the same way, by ministering to the whole person, especially via the soul. Actual treatment was extremely limited and going to the hospital often merely meant going to a place to find refuge. More frequently than not, the hospital meant a place in which to await death, especially for those who did not have the facilities to rest or die more comfortably at home.

In association with the main hospitals, there progressively developed more specialized institutions designed for segregating and housing particular classes of unfortunates – the lepers, the blind, the aged, the orphans. As the awareness of infection increased during the eighteenth century, these institutions were supplemented by the fever hospitals or pesthouses where patients were isolated in the hope of preventing them from spreading their disease to the community. All these trends intensified during the nineteenth century. To meet the ever increasing problems of crowd diseases, city hospitals grew into large professional institutions – centres of treatment enlarging on and replacing the medieval houses of mercy.

General acceptance of hospitalization by the public during the nineteenth century resulted in part from the control of hospital infections. Also, as scientific medicine advanced, only well-equipped institutions could provide the facilities required for new therapeutic procedures. By now, the intellectual mood had changed from that prevailing in the medieval houses of mercy. Scientific materialism had taken control of medicine. Disease was regarded as a derangement of the body machine; even mental illness was increasingly approached via the body.

Despite changes in public attitude, only a small percentage of patients, chiefly those with serious diseases, were hospitalized until the first decades of this century. Home care remained the general rule; the compassion and personal attention of the family physician still constituted the most common form of healing. The structure of medicine changed radically at the end of the nineteenth century when modern knowledge began to yield new methods of control for many kinds of bodily, and to some extent mental, derangement. At that time also, individual incomes were on the rise in the countries of Western civilization, and more and more people were taking out insurance coverage. A larger variety of patients could come to the hospital for care. No longer primarily an institution of mercy and a place where poor people went to die, the hospital progressively became a medical centre. Geared at first only for the treatment of disease, it eventually came to provide general guidance for the whole community in matters of health. The therapeutic innovations introduced during recent years are bound to change still further the philosophy of hospital management and of medical practice in general.

Until three decades ago, few therapies were really effective, and the main help to the patient was prolonged nursing care and alleviation of symptoms. Recovery from disease was slow; continued surveillance by the physician was needed at every step in order to meet emergencies. For this reason, the hospital was built, organized and administered on the assumption that the patient would be incapacitated for a long time and would be directly dependent on the medical staff for almost all aspects of his care. In contrast, many of the steps in diagnosis and even in therapy are now carried out by auxiliary personnel who, though functioning under the guidance of physicians, act in a certain measure on their own initiative. Furthermore, there has been a great acceleration in many types of medical procedures. Whether the patient comes within the domain of surgery, internal medicine, or any other speciality, the time for which hospitalization is mandatory is becoming shorter.

Another fact of importance in planning for the delivery of medical services is that a large percentage of illness is of a kind that does not take the patient to the hospital. The young physician going into practice soon discovers that most of his patients are troubled by conditions he had little chance to recognize, let alone treat, during his hospital training. Since the kinds of patients who find their way into hospitals provide an incomplete and distorted picture of the total health problems in a community, attempts are being made to extend the ministration of hospital medicine to the home, the school, the office, the shop and the factory. A hospital can encompass the whole range of the medical problems prevalent in a community only if the scope of its ministrations is broadened and enlarged conceptually. Modern societies must create a new type of medical instiution that might be called a hospital without walls.

Another phenomenon of our times that is changing the social approach to the prevention and treatment of disease is the increasing partnership between the medical profession and the other professions that also play a vital role in the health fields. Until recently medicine concerned itself exclusively with the care of the sick, a highly personal relation between the healer and the individual patient. This role is as important today as it ever was, but other fundamentally medical social problems, which yet transcend traditional medical activities, have arisen.

As technology invades more and more of our existence, it generates pathological states affecting the public as a whole, and demanding collective action. In this sense, a new need is rapidly emerging: the necessity for a science of disease control and health management having contact with other social and technological specialities.

The health fields now depend so heavily on complex technical procedures and relate to so many different social activities that they can no longer be the monopoly of the health professions; they require the services of many other specialized skills. Collaboration between the health professions and other specialities will grow more urgent and more intimate as our society demands that steps be taken not only to treat its diseases but also to protect its health against the dangers created by technological innovations.

Physicians must learn to work with engineers, architects and general biologists, as well as with city planners, lawyers and politicians responsible for the management of our social life. Only through such collaboration can they help society ward off, insofar as it is possible, dangers to physical and mental health inherent in all technological and social changes, especially when these occur as rapidly as they do now. From urban renewal to safety measures in industry, from environmental pollution to the trial of new drugs and therapeutic procedures, the sociomedical problems are countless and require technical, legal and ethical consideration.

Unless the health professions take a vigorous stand in this

collaborative venture, they may well be gradually edged out of many social aspects of their activities. The danger of such a prospect is that persons trained exclusively or primarily in the physical and social sciences often find it difficult to comprehend all the complexities of the issues involved in health problems. Technical knowledge must be supplemented by a broad understanding of man's nature, lest limited points of view generate oversimplified formulas of action. This broad view of man's welfare is peculiarly the province of the physician; indeed, his guidance is essential for the health of our technological world.

Many attempts are being made to incorporate in the new medical centres the attributes of both the medieval houses of mercy and the more recent hospitals. Ideally these classical attributes should be supplemented with the specialized services, teaching programmes and research activities linking modern medical practice to the various biomedical and social sciences. The medical centre should thus recapture the intimate relationship symbolized by the traditional picture of the family physician; it should cultivate the rational approach to disease that has grown out of scientific medicine; and it should be a forum for social studies where problems of the body, aspirations of the soul and needs of society are integrated into a new science of human and social engineering.

Two independent forces have completely revolutionized the scientific basis of medicine during the past century. Their result has been a trend away from concern with the individual patient toward a more impersonal approach to the problems of disease. One force in this trend is the increasing emphasis on the pathological and biochemical lesions of the sick person rather than on his responses to the total environment. Medical and surgical practices depend more and more on information derived from laboratory methods focused on the study of isolated histological structures and physiological functions. The second force in this trend is the development of public health programmes focused on the population as a whole. Whether he deals with waterborne infections, working conditions or environmental pollution, the public health officer concerns himself less and less with the art of medicine or with individual human beings; he functions as a biotechnologist rather than as a compassionate healer.

It is said that the personal physicians of the ancient Chinese were paid to keep their clients healthy rather than to cure them. In a similar way, through taxes and insurance, we pay physicians, nurses, scientists and the employees of multifarious government agencies to provide us with sanitation and vaccinations, advise us on what to eat or how to behave, and to watch over us for any sign of disease. Public and private funds in ever increasing amounts are being devoted to preventive measures designed to protect the health of the public.

The process of democratization and socialization is much less advanced in therapeutic than in preventive medicine. Highly dependent on personal physician-patient relationships, the practice of therapeutic medicine is not readily converted into mass practice; physicians must still spend much time on individual patients. Whereas the prevention of disease can often be achieved at low cost, therapeutic medicine increasingly involves the use of expensive techniques, equipment and supplies.

The constant increase in the cost of individualized medical care does not mean greater financial rewards to physicians and nurses. Nor does it stem from inefficiency in the management of hospitals. The cost increases because medicine now provides new kinds of highly complex and costly services. Therapeutic medicine is probably now entering a phase of medically diminishing returns. Many of its most spectacular and costly achievements are of help to only a few. Procedures such as open-heart surgery, the maintenance of patients with so-called artificial kidneys, and the control of phenylketonuria, constitute great technological feats, but they benefit only a minute percentage of the population while they loom very large on the national budget for health.

Economic considerations are in principle irrelevant to the right of every human being to health. Partly in consideration of this philosophy, almost every aspect of disease control is everywhere rapidly becoming a responsibility of government, whatever the political philosophy in power. Contrary to what is generally believed, the universal trend to make the care of the sick a collective rather than an individual responsibility is not fundamentally new. In the past only a few people could afford the services of private physicians. Religious and other benevolent organizations were then responsible for most medical care. What is new is the universal acceptance of the social philosophy that the prevention of disease is the responsibility of government rather than the responsibility of private groups.

While modern medicine must be based on the kind of scientific knowledge that permits generalizations about *Homo sapiens*, this knowledge is rarely sufficient to account for the medical problems of a particular person. For one thing, each person converts experiences and events into symbols in a highly individual manner and reacts to these symbols as though they were actual stimuli. For another, even when he professes to be an uncompromising rationalist, man is always influenced by irrational thoughts. Preoccupations that transcend plain material existence are as deeply ingrained in man's nature as is the way he uses his hands or digests his food. Psychic forces often determine the character and intensity of man's responses to the environment. Although imaginings, fears and hopes cannot be readily described, let alone quantified, these forces are no less significant in the causation and control of disease than are the structures and reactions measured by physical and chemical methods. William Osler had these complexities in mind when he said, 'It is more important to know what sort of patient has a disease than what sort of a disease a patient has.'

In all societies at all times, physicians have exploited, consciously or unconsciously, the fact that body ailments can be mollified by influencing the mind. Equivalent in Europe to the impressive appearance and incantations of ancient medicine men were the dark frock coat of the physician a few generations ago, his gold-headed cane and his dignified carriage. The modern physician has at his command powerful remedies and has given up these props, but he cultivates nevertheless a certain kind of bedside manner that contributes to his therapeutic effectiveness. He still believes with Alan Gregg that 'a miraculous moment comes when the doctor himself becomes the treatment'.

Although the trend toward the impersonal approach to disease control based on physicochemical biology will certainly continue, it can be predicted that certain aspects of human medicine will remain largely intuitive and highly personal. In this regard, human medicine will remain different from veterinary medicine. The professional attitude of the physician does not have its basis only in the natural sciences; it is conditioned by peculiarities of man's nature, especially by humanistic and ethical considerations that give a unique value to each human being.

Social Determinants of Biomedical Control

In most cases genetic endowment and racial origin play only a small role in determining the types and severity of the diseases most prevalent in a particular region or a particular social group. Whether they be of African, American Indian, European or Oriental origin, and whatever the complexity of their racial mixtures, human populations usually acquire the burden of diseases characteristic of the geographical area and of the social group in which they are born and live.

Medically speaking, man is more the product of his environment than of his genetic endowment. The health of human beings is determined not by their race but by the conditions under which they live.

So crucial are social factors in the causation and control of disease that it seems worthwhile to consider briefly a few illustrations of the complex interplay between economic conditions, the health of the people, and biomedical knowledge. Diseases caused by scarcity deserve first consideration because they are so widespread and have such tragic consequences in the underdeveloped parts of the world.

Malnutrition unquestionably underlies a large percentage of the disease problems in underdeveloped countries. In most cases, shortages of food and bad nutritional habits grow out of economic limitations and unwise traditional practices, both social factors. We might expect to find the solution to problems of malnutrition in political and social reforms rather than in the acquisition of more scientific knowledge. Actually, both approaches are equally essential. To be effective, political and social measures must be based on sophisticated scientific information concerning nutritional needs, the chemical constitution of foodstuffs, and the agricultural potentialities of the land.

Nutritional surveys have revealed that deficiencies in protein intake and in the absorption of certain vitamins constitute a far more frequent cause of severe malnutrition than do shortages of calories. Since malnutrition rarely results primarily from undernutrition, it cannot be corrected merely by producing more food. What is needed is the development of diets with the proper chemical composition. Since certain mixtures of foodstuffs, made up chiefly of plant products, can provide a correct balance of all essential nutrients, nutritional formulas favourable to health and compatible with the economies of developing countries should be possible.

Chemical knowledge, however pertinent, cannot define the kind of food that will be readily accepted by the people and therefore beneficial to them. In each region and each culture a number of food habits that take an immense amount of effort to change predominate. At the end of the First World War corn (maize) was shipped by the American Relief Committee to the famished people of Europe; Europeans were unable to use this particular kind of grain because it was foreign to their nutritional traditions, so much so that they did not even know how to cook it and incorporate it in their diets. Knowledge of the chemical composition of foods and their theoretical nutritional value must be supplemented by know-how in production methods and a sophisticated awareness of what is socially acceptable in a given region.

Among other complications, human beings often develop physiological adjustments to nutritional scarcity and acquire food habits and other behaviour patterns unfavourable to health and to social growth. Recent physiological and behavioural studies have revealed that these adjustments to undernutrition or malnutrition have distant consequences of far-reaching importance. People born and raised in an environment where food intake is quantitatively or qualitatively inadequate seem to achieve a certain form of physiological adaptation to low food intake. Unconsciously, they tend to restrict their physical and mental activity to reduce their nutritional needs; they become adjusted to undernutrition or malnutrition by living less intensely. Physical and mental apathy and other forms of indolence have long been assumed to have a racial or climatic origin. These behavioural traits often constitute instead a form of physiological adjustment to nutritional deficiencies, particularly if these have been experienced early in life.

Indolence resulting from adaptation to an inadequate food intake has obvious merits for survival under conditions of scarcity; indolence has even some romantic appeal for the harried and tense observer or tourist arriving from a competitive society. The dismal aspect of metabolic and mental adjustment to undernutrition or malnutrition is that it creates a vicious circle. Populations that have been nutritionally deprived during early life may remain healthy as long as no important effort is required of them, but they commonly exhibit little resistance to stress. They are often unwilling, probably because they find it difficult, to make the efforts required to improve their economic status. Statesmen who attempt to stimulate national economies often encounter a baffling lassitude stemming from prolonged nutritional deprivation.

Little is known of the physiological mechanisms of adaptation to nutritional scarcity. Ignorance in this field is so great that nutritionists would be hard put to correct the effects of early food deprivation even if they could find methods for providing an optimum diet to adults in deprived populations. The production of more food and better food is a technological and social problem; the improvement of nutritional status demands in addition sophisticated biomedical knowledge.

The control of diarrheal diseases constitutes another problem in which social action is likely to fail unless guided by scientific understanding of etiology. Since infectious processes certainly play an important role in most kinds of intestinal disorders, it has been commonly assumed that their medical control should be based on the widespread distribution of drugs and vaccines against intestinal pathogens. Contrary to supposition, the etiology of diarrheal diseases is not at all understood. Prophylactic and therapeutic measures based on such inadequate knowledge are seldom useful and do more harm than good in many cases. General dietary improvement, better practices of infant feeding and handling, or even simply an abundant supply of clean water are probably far more effective and less costly approaches to the control of many intestinal disorders than management with drugs and vaccines.

Both malnutrition and diarrheal diseases create medical problems especially in the young age groups. These disorders account for a large percentage of infant mortality among destitute populations. Their importance for the communities involved greatly transcends the problems revealed by infant mortality statistics. Children who have suffered nutritional deficiencies or prolonged infectious processes during the early stages of their development commonly fail to develop into healthy, vigorous adults. The pathological experiences of early life tend to depress physical and mental activity during youth and the teenage period, and very frequently the unfavourable effects persist throughout adulthood and appear irreversible.

Malnutrition and infection are not the only disadvantageous early experiences generating irreversible pathological effects. Lasting damage is a frequent consequence of most physiological, emotional or social forms of early deprivation. Some of the nefarious effects exerted by early influences are so lasting that they condition most activities during the whole life-span with an attendant effect on the social and economic performance of the society. Control of disease during the early phases of life and guidance of all aspects of physical and mental development during youth may constitute the most far-reaching and useful methods for improving health, especially in underdeveloped countries.

In this light, the extent of health improvement to be expected from building ultramodern hospitals with highly trained staffs and up-to-date equipment is probably trivial compared with results from the much lower cost of providing infants and children with well-balanced food, sanitary conditions and a stimulating environment. Acceptance of this thesis would imply profound changes in medicosocial policies and would affect also the selection of problems in scientific research. Old people deserve our help and sympathy, and adults constitute the resources of the present, but the young represent the future. Much biomedical knowledge and social wisdom is needed to determine comparative degrees of emphasis in the medical care of different age groups.

We have been concerned so far with diseases that are especially prevalent and destructive in underprivileged populations. The common diseases of prosperous industrialized countries could have served just as well to illustrate the need for biomedical guidance in social planning.

As we have seen, chronic and degenerative diseases of adult life in prosperous countries involve many factors. Obscurity still surrounds the precise mechanisms relating the increased incidence of chronic and degenerative diseases to industrial environment and urban ways of life. Assuming deficiencies in etiological understanding, some general findings of the relation of social health to the total environment make the problem relevant to all countries of the world, regardless of their state of economic development.

Industrialization and urbanization will soon become almost universal. In view of the speed at which social and technological changes occur, many of the environmental stresses common in the affluent countries today are likely to spread to the rest of the world in the very near future. Unless carefully anticipated and controlled, these disturbances will add their deleterious effects to those of malnutrition and such infectious diseases as tuberculosis, malaria or schistosomiasis; they will create new kinds of physiological misery in the areas of the world undergoing industrialization.

The health problems posed by social and technologic changes cannot be predicted with confidence because they have determinants peculiar to each area and to each community. Smogs differ in composition according to the climate, the topography of the district, the type of technological operation and the kind of fuel used. Similarly, each industrial process engenders its own class of occupational dangers and water pollution. Clearly then, public health problems caused by rapid industrial growth cannot be solved by slavishly applying control methods developed under other conditions. Solutions will require programmes of research and control suited to the peculiarities of local situations.

Even more important, the 'diseases of civilization' will not be auotmatically eliminated by improving the economic status, since they are created by industrial growth. Just as scientific guidance is required for the control of the diseases of scarcity prevailing at present in underdeveloped regions, so a new kind of science must be created to deal with the medical problems affecting industrial areas that could properly be called *maldeveloped*. Unless the social structure can be managed on the basis of suitable biomedical knowlelge, all countries in the process of becoming industrialized will soon duplicate the horrible conditions prevailing now in polluted, congested and inhuman industrial centres. It would be tragic indeed if technologic and economic growth meant the replacement of the diseases of scarcity by the diseases of affluence.

Ideally, the approach to disease control should be the same in all countries of the world, prosperous or underdeveloped. In practice, social and economic factors condition not only the incidence and manifestations of the various types of

disease but also the extent to which medical knowledge can use-
fully be applied to their control. Each society must therefore
have its own system of medicine and public health suited to
its particular needs and to its resources.

It might be assumed that the most rapid and effective way
to improve the medical situation in an emerging country would
be to introduce trained personnel from more developed areas.
Unfortunately the world's capital of physicians, scientists,
teachers and technicians is far too small to permit their export
in numbers sufficient to have a significant effect.

Fortunately, the practical impossibility of large-scale transfer of specialists and technical knowledge becomes less alarming when the medical needs of the emerging countries are
formulated not in the abstract but with regard to dominant
disease patterns. The most urgent need of the emerging countries is the control of nutritional and microbial diseases, a
problem best handled through relatively inexpensive collective methods of preventive medicine. Individual human beings
have the same unique value and dignity everywhere, but with
such limited natural and personnel resources, poor countries
would seem wise to focus their medical efforts at first on the
collective aspects of preventive medicine. If such is the case,
the development of medical services in the emerging countries
might parallel their economic evolution.

The first stage in the change from primitive patterns of disease control in a country undergoing industrialization might
be to introduce measures not customarily regarded as pertaining to health, programmes such as the development of
roads, bridges, telephones and dams, and the irrigation of farm-
land. Increased production and better distribution of food
is commonly the most essential need for health improvement.
Furthermore, the ability to reach a remote area rapidly over
good roads and to span long distances by telephone is often
critical in stamping out an epidemic or overcoming famine in
a local area.

The second stage of development would be more medical
than the first stage, though not on a personal level. It would

consist of measures designed to bring about environmental changes directly related to disease control. General sanitary improvements such as draining swamps or large-scale spraying of residual insecticides contribute materially to the management of insect-borne diseases.

The third stage would introduce a more personal relationship but one having a noncontinuing character. Examples would be immunization programmes implemented every two or three years in remote villages, or elementary training in sanitary or nutritional practices of selected members of a tribe. The men who deliver biomedical technology establish some personal contact with the local population but are not expected to be on call or to return soon.

These three stages depend upon collective methods rather than personal physician-patient relationships for the application of biomedical sciences. The personal approach to disease control, common in Western civilizations, would represent an entirely different kind of medical action and create in the recipient public hopes and eventually demands possible to meet only through a far more costly type of medical organization.

In the fourth stage, the community would assume that individuals are entitled to medical care on a continuing basis, whether this care meets a real biological need or is merely a response to a personal demand. Such personal service might be paid for on a cash basis, through insurance programmes or by government agencies, but the purely financial aspects are irrelevant here. What matters is that moving into this fourth stage constitutes a crucial and probably irreversible step. It is crucial because personal medicine has a low economic return compared with collective preventive measures. It constitutes therefore a heavy financial burden for any society trying to lift itself by its bootstraps. It is irreversible because of the new emotional attitudes it creates. When a baby dies in a primitive village, the mother naturally grieves the loss, but she accepts it as one of life's inescapable tragedies. Once she has discovered that a physician can save babies from death, she will regard society's failure to make the resources of modern medicine available to her baby an act of social injustice or even of deliberate cruelty.

The fifth stage involves medicine as practised by physicians belonging to or in direct contact with a modern medical centre. Ideally in this situation the physician assimilates as fast as possible all the new contributions of biomedical sciences and applies them to the health problems of individuals.

The various stages outlined above do not follow each other in orderly sequence. They will overlap, and their concrete expression will retain traits peculiar to the societies in which they occur. Culturally disparate systems of medicine do co-exist everywhere in the world. In the most highly developed countries, countless human beings whose survival depends on the federal, state and city systems of preventive medicine resort to medical healers in whom they have faith, religious or otherwise, for most of the ailments from which they suffer. The medicine man in the Indian reservation has his counterpart on Main Street, Broadway and Park Avenue all over the United States and in all the most sophisticated cities of Western civilization.

Every type of human society develops the kind of medicine it can afford and the practices that suit its cultural traditions. Only biomedical science can provide the knowledge required for policies of collective medical control necessary for survival in the modern world.

Potentialities of Disease Control

Like all eighteenth-century social reformers, Benjamin Franklin had absolute faith in the power of science to solve human problems. In a letter to the chemist Joseph Priestley, he prophesied that the time would come when 'all diseases may by sure means be prevented or cured, not excepting that of old age'. Although the medical utopia envisaged by Franklin has not yet come into being, there is a large element of truth in his prediction; many of the most destructive diseases of his time have now been brought under control in prosperous countries. Franklin himself would probably be surprised that it took less than two centuries of experimental science to convert into realities some of the boldest medical imaginings of the Age of Reason.

Biomedical technology has become so effective during the past few decades that one can anticipate the possibility of manipulating at will some of the most important aspects of man's nature. The transplantation of organs, for example, may soon become commonplace; the purely surgical aspects of this problem have been solved, and rapid progress is being made toward the development of techniques for overcoming the tissue incompatibilities that have so far prevented the survival of organs transferred from one person to another. Several medical scientists have even suggested that higher apes be selected and raised with the purpose of supplying suitable spare parts for the human body.

Other scientists believe that the development of completely artificial contrivances will prove in the long run more useful and practical than a programme of organ transplantation. Electrical pacesetters for the heart and external dialysis as a partial substitute for renal function (the so-called artificial kidney) have already found a place in orthodox medical management. The success experienced in the use of artificial heart valves and arterial walls may open the way to constructing plastic prostheses of heart or kidney that would remain functional in the human body.

Endless also are the possibilities on the horizon for modifying the human brain and controlling behaviour. The administration of various hormones, prenatal and early postnatal manipulations, and surgical or psychological methods akin to those used for surgical lobotomy or for brainwashing are but a few of the techniques that might be used to alter the personality, in either a permanent or a reversible manner. Even the hereditary endowment of man may soon become amenable to wilful alteration.

The few examples mentioned have been selected at random from among many others merely to illustrate the wide range of methods modern medical science can call into play for the treatment of disease through manipulations of the body and the mind. The application of these methods to disease control offers such diversified potentialities that one can anticipate scientific solutions for almost any medical problem, once it has been clearly defined. However, the theoretical possibility of solving a disease problem is no guarantee that society will or can make the practical efforts needed to find the solution or will convert scientific knowledge into practical action. In many cases the greatest limitations to disease control arise not from lack of scientific knowledge or of technical methods for its application but from economic and social constraints.

While the scientific method is immensely effective for dealing with the technical aspects of biomedical problems, it provides little or no guidance in deciding what should be done among all the things that could be done; by its nature it is constrained from relating technical solutions to the fundamental needs of man and his societies. While there are no foreseeable limits to the theoretical possibilities of scientific medicine, economic, social and ethical difficulties often complicate or prevent altogether the practical utilization of existent knowledge for the prevention and treatment of disease.

Economic Limitations to Disease Control

Economic considerations naturally affect the percentage of individual and national income devoted to medical care. In the United States medical expenditure rose from 3·3 per cent of the gross national product in 1929 to 4.5 per cent in 1933 and fell again in the late 1930s. While the gross national product was reduced by almost half during the profound and prolonged economic depression, expenditure on medical care dropped by less than a third. The proportion of its income that a given community spends on medical care seems to vary within much narrower limits than the proportion devoted to other items in the budget. Even more remarkable, all the developed countries spend about the same percentage of their national income on medical care, no matter how this is financed. The official figures in 1953 ranged from 3.76 per cent for the Netherlands to 4·56 per cent for New Zealand. For most other countries of Western civilization, the percentage has consistently hovered slightly above 4 per cent during the past two decades.

Even under optimum conditions, the present programmes for prevention and treatment of disease are grossly inadequate. According to an official statement, the National Health Survey now being carried out by the U.S. Public Health Service has revealed that in 1964,

eight out of ten noninstitutionalized persons aged 65 or over had one or more chronic conditions. Some of these, of course, are minor (allergies, bronchitis, and the like), but many others involve serious illnesses such as heart disease, arthritis, and diabetes. The activity of more than half the aged with chronic conditions is limited to some extent. When these figures are projected against the anticipated 22 million older persons in the population of 1975, the challenge to the health professions is staggering.[1]

Every single day in the United States more than 1,000 new persons are added to the rank of the 18 million (in 1966) who are older than 65 years of age. More than 11,000 persons 100 years old or older are now drawing Social Security benefits. Gratifying as it is to know of new medical procedures permitting prolongation of life, it is frightening to realize the extent to which each achievement adds to the medical load of the future. Even the wealthiest economies may not be able to carry forever the enormous burden created by the scientific advances that permit 'medicated survival'.

Although it is widely presumed that the growth of medical science and the development of health services will progressively reduce the number of persons requiring medical care, there is no evidence for this assumption. The experience gained from two decades of medicine under the National Health Service and the National Insurance Service in Great

1. John D. Porterfield, 'The Merchandising of Public Health', *New York Academy of Medicine Bulletin*, 1964, vol. 40, p. 131.

Britain show that, contrary to expectations, the cost of the national services has increased constantly from year to year.

Similar increases in medical expenditure have taken place in all the countries of Western civilization, no matter what the political system and the social methods for distributing medical services. In 1964 one out of every seven persons in the United States entered a hospital during the course of a year, as compared to one out of every eighteen thirty years ago. The percentage is constantly rising.

The increased demand for medical care reflects the higher standards of health that society demands as it becomes more sophisticated and prosperous and as medicine advances. Less encouraging is the probable danger of medical progress being outstripped by a real increase in the incidence of disease, or at least by a change in the pattern of diseases. To complicate the situation further, a larger percentage of the population now consists of persons in the older age groups.

A continually increasing demand for medical care can thus be expected to create eventually a debilitating drain on financial and technical resources, even in wealthy countries. Important in this regard, the practices of modern therapeutic medicine depend increasingly upon highly skilled persons with long, expensive and specialized training, men who must constantly undergo further education in order to keep in step with scientific advances. A scarcity of adequately trained personnel, rather than a shortage of funds, is likely to constitute the Achilles' heel of disease control in the future.

Standards of medical care are determined by a number of unrelated and entirely independent factors. There are minimum biological needs below which human beings or social groups cannot function effectively. The state of medical knowledge determines other needs. Experience has shown that the availability of new techniques of prevention and treatment increases the demand on the medical sciences by changing the criteria of health. Finally, the use of modern medical advances paradoxically creates new medical needs. Prolonging the life of the aged and of the sick increases the numbers of persons who constantly depend on costly care. More important, perhaps, medical advances create an atmosphere of rising expectations; human beings are no longer willing to tolerate even the mild physical disabilities to which all flesh is heir, once they become aware that pain and discomfort can be mollified.

As a significant contribution to the high cost of medical care, practically all forms of disease control now depend on a highly complex technology. This is true even in the case of simple drugs, whether they are used for the control of pain, infection or behaviour. The discovery of a drug is always the outcome of numerous laboratory operations perhaps relatively simple in a particular case but always costly in the aggregate because only a small percentage of the substances tested are ever used. To illustrate, something less than one out of 20,000 substances tested for the prevention or treatment of malaria have proved of practical value in the control of this disease.

Safety tests are becoming an ever more significant cost item in the development and use of drugs. Before any new drug can be released to physicians, it must be tested for toxicity on several animal species; these tests must be carried out for prolonged periods of time, indeed for the whole life-span of that animal, because many deleterious effects manifest themselves only very slowly and under special conditions; finally, extensive and careful observations in human beings must precede approval by control agencies. The cost of testing for toxicity alone now amounts to many million dollars per drug, and this one item of production costs will continue to increase as safety requirements justifiably become more exacting.

Surgical operations on blood vessels, on the heart, on the brain or on the kidneys provide striking illustrations of the technological complexities involved in the achievements of modern medicine. The surgical act itself demands great knowledge and skill on the part of the surgeon and his assistants, but this represents only one aspect, and not the most costly, of the total operation. The more vital the organ involved, the more essential and complex are the accessory procedures required to maintain the physiological activities of the person before, during and after surgery. Physiological control always demands the use of elaborate mechanical and chemical apparatus, each one of which must be handled by scientific and technical personnel trained to a high degree of specialization.

Until the middle of the present century the medical profession was made up essentially of the physician, the surgeon and the nurse. Increasingly, different kinds of technologists, each with specialized equipment having a rapid rate of obsolescence, are supplementing the original core.

Changes in the technology of medical care have been so rapid and so profound that it is not yet possible to evaluate properly their consequences with regard to cost and personnel requirements. That our societies can afford to give to all those in need of medical help the total benefits of up-to-date medical science seems dubious. The time is rapidly approaching when medical ethics will have to be reformulated in the harsh light of economics.

Economic limitations will soon apply not only in the application of known methods of disease control but also in the acquisition of new theoretical and practical knowledge. We have witnessed during the past three decades a phenomenal increase in the financial support of medical research; in the United States the support from federal sources alone has gone from $50 million per year in 1940 to $1·2 billion (thousand million) in 1965. According to a recent official statement, expenditures for medical research have risen in the United States from about 5.6 per cent to 8.8 per cent of all research and development. In absolute terms, the growth has been even more impressive: from about $160 million in 1950 to an estimated $1·8 billion in 1965. This represents an escalation of effort to improve the human condition, drawing on all sectors of the economy – government, industry and philanthropy. Although some further increase can be expected, the consensus is that soon a ceiling will be reached. When this happens, those supporting medical science will have to choose what kinds of research are to be emphasized and what kinds must be neglected. To give adequate support to all worthy projects simultaneously will certainly become impossible.

Fields of medical research that bear, directly or indirectly, on the often fatal adult and senile degenerative diseases receive the most generous support at present. It might be argued that mental retardation and disturbances of behaviour in childhood are more important in the long run because they affect the future of our societies.

Even as limited a question as the technical problems posed by production of antiviral vaccines can create social dilemmas. The theoretical aspects of vaccine production are now essentially solved. While it is possible in principle to produce vaccines against almost any type of virus disease, the technical development of such vaccines, especially the safety testing, requires an enormous amount of highly skilled effort. With several hundred strains of viruses known to cause disease in man, the development of all possible vaccines is entirely impractical. Where, then, should emphasis be placed? On viral infections that produce tragic disabilities, such as paralysis, but affect only a small percentage of the population? Or on the viral infections with much less dramatic effects, such as the common respiratory diseases, that affect most of the population and lie behind much of the absenteeism from school, office, factory or the armed services?

Medical research could in theory find a scientific solution for most of the disease problems of our times. There are not, and cannot be, enough resources or scientific skills to attack all the problems that cry out for solution or to apply all the theoretical knowledge that has been developed. The question will be what of all the things that could be done should be done. In all cases these decisions will involve criteria that transcend scientific knowledge and judgement. They will have to be made on the basis of social and ethical values.

Some Ethical Dilemmas of Modern Medicine

Fifty years ago the physician, like the engineer, could approach his task with the confidence that he was acting as a benefactor of mankind. The situation has now changed. Nuclear warfare, industrial fumes and automobile casualties have made it obvious that the beneficial aspects of the engineer's skill have their destructive counterparts. Difficult as it is to imagine, medical action can also have undesirable consequences; there is no doubt that medical technology also creates situations that threaten the welfare of mankind.

The techniques of modern medicine are so powerful, so far-reaching and often so indiscriminate that they can menace the health of future generations even as they save the lives of today's patients. They can damage human personality even as they improve the functions of the body machine. Physicians have always known that the practice of medicine poses difficult ethical problems. Although the Hippocratic Oath has been accepted as a code of medical conduct for two and a half thousand years, the exact formulation of medical ethics is still a much disputed subject.

Everyone agrees that scientific knowledge and technical competence are not sufficient for the practice of medicine. The quality of the service rendered by a doctor to his patients reflects both his personal integrity and that attribute designated by classical scholars as 'caritas'.

Medical ethics is concerned primarily with the trust placed by the patient in his doctor and involves moral judgements. The professional and ethical responsibilities of the physician are not limited to the patient entrusted to his care; they extend to the society in which he lives and to mankind in general. At times, the good of society is in conflict with the patient's demand. Notification of certain infectious diseases is an imperative practice, whatever inconvenience it may cause to the patient. Saving the life of a patient with a genetic disease is likely to encourage the spread of the deleterious genes through the community. Thus the welfare of the individual patient is often incompatible with the general interest. Since deciding between what is right and what is wrong involves value judgements, the relation of medical ethics to the public weal is by necessity ill-defined. Most medical situations are socially and ethically complex, and for this reason it is desirable that judges of professional conduct be persons experienced both in the law and in the art of medicine.

The possibility of unlimited progress toward an unattainable medical utopia becomes even more painful as we approach the ideal of a classless society. Whatever the income of a nation and however effective its medical establishment, some medical procedures can never be made available to all those who need them, simply because of the shortage of technical skills. Yet the concept of a two-class society is even more repugnant medically than it is from the economic point of view. Human ethics demands that the unskilled workman and the bank president be given the same medical privileges. Unless unexpected scientific developments truly revolutionize medical practice by making it far less costly and far more simple technically than it now is, past and present ethical principles will have to be reformulated in the light of inescapable social limitations.

The possibility of postponing death in every age group, another consequence of technological progress, creates further ethical problems for the medical conscience. To save the life of a child suffering from some hereditary defect is a humane act which affords great professional gratification; its long-range consequence is commonly to magnify the medical problems of the future. Likewise, prolonging the life of an aged and ailing person must be weighed against the possible hardships that medicated survival entails for this very person, for his family and for the community. Such ethical problems are not new, but they were rarely encountered so starkly in the past when the physician's power of action was so limited. They are bound to become more frequent and more disturbing as physicians become more able to prolong biological existence. Human beings who can derive neither profit nor pleasure from life and whose survival creates large social problems in terms of emotional tension or economic burden (usually both) pose questions of major ethical import to physicians.

By postponing death from irreversible physical and mental defects, we allow the accumulation in our communities of persons who need continuous and exacting medical supervision. By making physical life almost effortless and by minimizing exposure to infection and inclemencies, we reduce the opportunity for those adaptive reactions that would otherwise increase the resistance of the body and the mind to the unavoidable accidents and challenges of life. Medical science now makes it possible for almost every newborn infant to survive, however defective he may be and whatever the inadequacies of his hereditary endowment. Admittedly, genetic defects and physiological deficiencies need not be a serious handicap in a society equipped to correct their manifestations. An acute dilemma will arise when the accumulation of the weak and the sick constitute an economic and medical burden difficult to manage even in prosperous and dedicated societies.

Equally disturbing are the ethical problems posed by the use of medical procedures unquestionably beneficial to society yet dangerous for the individual. Such a situation is illustrated by the use of certain vaccines. There is no doubt that vaccination against smallpox has been so effective that this disease has been almost eliminated from certain parts of the world. Smallpox vaccine does produce serious encephalitis in a few persons even when it is administered with the utmost care. The chance of contracting smallpox is now so slight in our communities that, paradoxically enough, the risk of accidents originating from the vaccine is much greater than the chance of contracting the disease itself. For this reason, many persons naturally advocate that the practice of general vaccination be abandoned. It is certain, though, that smallpox would once more become a public threat if a large percentage of the population failed to be vaccinated. Freedom from smallpox must be paid for in the form of a few deaths resulting from vaccination of the public. In many other similar situations, the health of the general public depends upon the willingness of its individual members to accept some inconveniences and take a few risks.

Experimentation on man is usually an indispensable final step in the discovery of new therapeutic procedures or drugs, creating another perplexing problem of medical ethics. Studies in animals can go far toward developing safe surgical techniques and demonstrating the efficacy and safety of drugs. The first surgeons who operated on the lungs, the heart or the brain were by necessity experimenting on man, since knowledge derived from animal experimentation is never entirely applicable to the human species. Similarly, many drugs found safe in animals can produce toxic effects in human beings – witness the thalidomide tragedy.

The U.S. Food and Drug Administration legitimately imposes increasingly elaborate safety tests on the release of drugs for use in clinical practice in that country. This restricting policy is not without its drawbacks. It interferes with the development of new drugs and probably prevents the use of some drugs that might be helpful under certain conditions. It is now realized that all the drugs introduced during the past three decades can under certain conditions cause severe toxic effects and even death, both in animals and in men. This is true of drugs absolutely essential to the modern practice of medicine; for example penicillin and cortisone. Had their potential toxicity been recognized, several of our most useful drugs would probably have been rejected early in the course of safety tests.

Conflicts between medical progress and medical ethics appear in almost all aspects of the science and practice of medicine. The physician or surgeon who decides to use a new drug or therapeutic procedure in handling a disease for which an accepted treatment already exists is experimenting on man; he can be sued for malpractice even though his action was justified according to his best medical judgement. Thus, a strict and legalistic interpretation of medical ethics almost invariably stands in the way of medical progress. This state of affairs is not peculiar to medicine; it applies just as well to other types of technological innovations; all new technologies involve dangers that cannot be entirely foreseen. Thoughtful men must of necessity be concerned with safety, but societies can continue to grow only if they are willing to take calculated risks. In medicine, as in technology and all other aspects of life, precautionary measures are needed for survival, but excessive concern for safety can result in social paralysis.

The Manipulation of Man's Biological Future

Men have tried throughout history to direct biological evolution by various social practices, such as selecting mates with desirable physical and mental attributes or creating a caste system. The genetic effects thus obtained are usually of little consequence. Master races of famous families differ from other social classes less by virtue of their genetic endowment than because they derive biological advantages from their ways of life. So-called blue-blood characteristics are in most cases the expressions of the social environment and the conditions of early upbringing, not manifestations of genetic superiority. Mankind's evolutionary development so far has been largely unpremeditated; it has been the outcome of complex and uncontrolled interplays between man's nature and environmental factors.

The methods of modern medicine may eventually exert a much deeper influence on the genetic constitution of mankind than have all the conscious efforts of the past. Through its influence on the rate of population increase, in addition to the probable deleterious effects of its ability to save genetically defective children, modern medicine will indirectly affect the future of the human race. Let it first be clear that, contrary to general belief, medical advances are not solely responsible for the population avalanche. The largest population increases are occurring in some of the most economically backward countries without benefit of sanitation or of medical services. Many different social forces accelerate population growth. More efficient means of transportation and communication have decreased the number of deaths from famines; or again, technological innovations have recently made available for human settlement vast areas that used to be desert and therefore uninhabitable.

Medical advances have influenced population growth chiefly by reducing death rates among children and young adults in certain areas of the world. The control of mosquitoes, lice and flies by DDT and other insecticides has lowered considerably the incidence of insect-borne diseases, especially malaria; vaccination has reduced the ravages of smallpox and a few other viral infections; the widespread use of isoniazid seems to be partially checking the spread of tuberculosis. It is not easy to estimate the cumulative effect of all these procedures, but there is no doubt that together they are saving the lives of large numbers of young people. The distressing consequence of this achievement is that instead of dying rapidly of infection, more and more children are now condemned to suffer from malnutrition and to live in squalor.

If the various birth and death rates were to remain at their present levels, the increase in world population would become catastrophic within less than a century. In the past, industrialization, urbanization and a decrease in infant mortality have usually resulted in a rapid lowering of birth rates. On the basis of this experience, we can hope that along with the possibility of saving the young from death the prospects of a more abundant and hopeful life will provide an atmosphere favourable for the limitation of family size through birth control. This trend will probably be accelerated by the development of improved contraceptive techniques.

Family planning, however, is likely to create new biological problems which are little if at all understood. Once infant mortality has been reduced to levels as low as those prevailing in prosperous countries, an average of three children per family is far too high for population control. Surprising as it may be, this family size results in a doubling of the population within a very few decades. The population can be stabilized only if the average number of children born per couple does not exceed 2·3. Such low birth rates would leave little room for the operation of the selective forces that have maintained the genetic characteristics of the human race in the past. In truth, little is known of these genetic aspects of the population problem, and it is not justified therefore to state that they spell disaster for the future of mankind. Nevertheless, the prospects are sufficiently alarming to render imperative and urgent a scientific study of medical and social methods of preventing genetic deterioration.

From the evidence, even in the healthiest societies, a large percentage of children are born with genetic defects inherited from their parents. The overall rate of mutation is more than likely being increased by certain factors ubiquitous in modern life, such as radiation, environmental pollutants, food additives or drugs. Finally, it is possible, although not convincingly proven, that new techniques of prophylaxis and therapy interfere with selective processes that depend on the weeding out of the unfit.

The fear that genetic self-correction may no longer operate is creating a renewal of scientific and popular interest in the problems of eugenics. Some geneticists claim that man can avoid genetic deterioration only if that approximate 20 per cent of the population who are heavily laden with genetic defects either fail to live until maturity or fail to reproduce. Increasingly, the proponents of eugenics go beyond advocating methods for preventing genetic deterioration. They claim that man could be positively improved physically and mentally if society were willing to favour the selective reproduction of the human gene types representing desirable qualities.

The dream of voluntary selective reproduction is not new. It can be traced back to Plato and to early sociologists who advocated caste systems. It was revived in a more modern form by Sir Francis Galton during the nineteenth century, but the techniques for converting the eugenic dream into reality are only now being developed. Methods for preserving reproductive cells in an active state are so dependable that frozen spermatozoa can remain viable and available in storage banks for indefinite periods of time; they can be utilized for artificial insemination long after the death of the donor. Preservation of the female ovum also looms as a possibility in the foreseeable future. Children, without doubt, can be produced at will from the reproductive cells of parents selected for certain desired genetic traits. Granted that artificial insemination is a practical possibility, the technical aspects of the problem constitute only the least perplexing of the many questions surrounding it.

Admittedly, artificial insemination has proved an effective practice in animal husbandry. In this case, well-defined goals account for its success. An animal breeder may want specifically to produce cows yielding more milk, or horses likely to win races. In contrast, there is no agreement on the ideal attributes of human beings. Opinions about the world and men change, and this necessarily complicates the selection of semen donors. No one disagrees to eliminating the gross physical and mental defects which afflict the human race, although even this limited approach poses problems of judgement and of execution far more complex than usually realized. The choice of the positive attributes to be fostered raises questions of a more subtle nature.

Our present ways of life may soon be antiquated, and the future may demand qualities undreamed of at the present time. For all we know, resistance to radiation, noise, crowding, intense light, and to the repetition of boring activities, may be essential for biological and social success in future civilizations. Who knows, furthermore, whether mankind is better served by persons who prize, above all, individuality and self-realization, or by those who regard service to the collective society as the highest form of life? One of the fundamental difficulties standing in the way of formulating eugenic programmes is that no one knows what men want to become. No two philosophers agree on what is the ideal form of human life.

Other difficulties come from the lack of basic knowledge concerning the genetic determinants of man's nature. Also, all important aspects of human life are profoundly affected by environmental factors, and these differ from one social group to another. Body size, physiological functions, learning ability and emotional attitudes are determined at least as much by the conditions of early life as by the genetic endowment.

Many biologists believe that mankind could be improved more effectively and more rapidly by controlling the environment than by altering the genetic constitution. Others claim that even better results could be achieved by modifying the course of man's development through manipulation of his physiological processes. Still others advocate the use of artificial contrivances capable of replacing or supplementing body structures. Mechanical hearts or kidneys and brains reshaped by prenatal or early postnatal interventions are among the prospects recently mentioned by eminent biologists.

Medical science is now contemplating the manipulation of man through biotechnological procedures that alter his very personality. Even at present, mental states can be influenced by many different techniques from yoga to hypnosis to drugs. In man as well as in animals, electric stimulations of particular areas in the brain can produce behavioural changes and even a sense of well-being in the whole organism. Similar effects can be produced by psychedelic drugs such as mescaline, lysergic acid diethylamide (LSD) and psilocybin. The knowledge derived from these practices is immensely exciting because it enlarges the understanding of the mechanisms through which the human mind operates, but by the same token it is also frightening because almost inevitably knowledge is used for control.

The question will eventually arise as to the identity of the person modified by biotechnology. What will be the legal, moral or psychiatric identity of a human being so altered by medical manipulation that he has become almost an artificial chimera? In the final analysis, one of the cruellest dilemmas of modern medicine is to decide which aspects of man's nature can be ethically tampered with and which ones should be respected at all costs.

The threat to mankind posed by the technologies derived from modern physicochemical and biological sciences gives a dramatic timeliness to Montaigne's admonition that 'Science without conscience is but death of the soul.' Modern medicine, in particular, is in the process of becoming so powerful that some of its methods have remote and indirect consequences reaching far beyond the purpose for which they were intended. Increasingly, the science and practice of medicine will have to take the future of mankind into consideration. Technical proficiency never was a sufficient criterion for the physician; and it is becoming even less so as his powers of action become greater. Problems of medical ethics are bound to increase in complexity and will have to be defined on the basis of a deeper understanding of the human condition. The development of a true science of man may well be the most urgent forerunner of the formulation of a philosophy of medicine.

6 The Cultural Values of Biomedical Sciences

Ancient Medicine and the Emergence of Culture

High on a ledge in the cavern of Les Trois-Frères in southern France, a Paleolithic artist of the High Magdalenian era some fifteen thousand years ago painted one of the oldest portraits of man. Dubbed 'The Sorcerer' by anthropologists, it resembles closely an eighteenth-century picture of a Siberian shaman with animal features and wearing antlers. Reminiscent also of an Indian medicine man in the American Southwest, the Magdalenian Sorcerer symbolizes the real and mystical power of all medicine men in primitive societies everywhere.

Shamans, witch doctors and medicine men differ in training and social functions from one primitive society to another, but all have certain features in common. Usually skilled and experienced in the healing arts, medicine men frequently know well the fields, the forests and the streams. From observation they understand the effects of weather conditions on plant and animal life, and as practical and spiritual leaders, they learn and transmit the history and myths of their tribe. Rites, chants and arts are the tools of their profession; with them they help their people to relate to their surroundings, to the forces of nature and to the various deities. In the course of time, by associating magical ceremonies with practical activities, medicine men often subconsciously correlate phenomena not obviously related. Little by little, such correlations enlarge the scope and bulk of their factual knowledge.

Certain anthropologists pragmatically define culture as an acquired or learned system of shared and transmitted ways enabling the cultural group to handle satisfactorily the problems of life. Other scholars define culture as the best that men have thought and known. Ancient medicine men embodied these two aspects of culture. The patterns of thought and life they developed referred to the practical aspects of material existence and became expressed in symbols and rites pleasurable to the people. From such factual and imaginative origins, the culture characteristics of each tribe progressively evolved and eventually became what we now call science and the humanities.

Medicine and the Natural Sciences

The infant first becomes aware of the world through subconscious processes; he organizes and rationalizes this awareness into systematic knowledge only later in life. And so it was for mankind as a whole. Naturally it is impossible to trace historically how observations and correlations at first subconscious and purely accidental were progressively transformed into conscious and systematic knowledge. That medicine reached this sophisticated state many thousands of years ago is certain. More impressive than their practical skills was the ability of ancient physicians to formulate large generalizations and to recognize cause-effect relationships between complex phenomena not obviously related. The view that the environment plays an important role in the problems of human biology, medicine and sociology has never been stated with greater breadth and clarity than it was at the dawn of science in the Hippocratic treatise, *Airs, Waters and Places*.

Ancient medicine also played a large and perhaps dominant role in the formulation of the methodology of experimental science. From medical practice, ancient physicians learned methods of diagnosis and the art of prognosis; they developed the habits and skills needed to organize objective knowledge in medicine and in other scientific fields. An intriguing characteristic of ancient medicine is that it incorporated most aspects of knowledge. Ancient physicians were concerned with the physiological effects of music, astronomical events, and religious beliefs, just as they were interested in anatomical structures, surgical techniques or the activities of drugs. Through the catholicism of their attitude, ancient medicine became the mother of the sciences, the inspiration of humanism, and the integrating force of culture.

Since the primary concern of medicine is man – in health and in disease, in happiness and in grief – it is not surprising that many physicians of all countries at all times have been writers and humanists. Equally true although less widely recognized, physicians have played a large role in the evolution of science until recent times. As late as the seventeenth century throughout Europe, perhaps especially in Italy, many of the great masters of the natural sciences were also practising physicians. Many of the most illustrious physicists, chemists and biologists of the nineteenth century (and not a few of the twentieth century) were trained as physicians; the questions that made them specialize in other fields of knowledge and discover the facts and laws of today's natural sciences were questions originally connected with their medical problems.

As knowledge increased, the various scientific specialities became more and more self-contained and independent of their medical origins. Medicine, which has for several thousand years provided the natural sciences with both philosophical inspiration and practical problems, has now abandoned its position of intellectual leadership. Since the middle of the nineteenth century the trend has been to regard scientific medical knowledge as a derivative of physics, chemistry, microbiology, genetics, psychology and other natural sciences. Two generations ago the enterprising medical scientist was likely to attempt becoming an expert in physiology or microbiology; more recently, he has become obsessed with biochemistry and molecular biology; soon he may attempt to master the fields of electronics and communication theory. Once the generator of natural sciences, medicine is gradually becoming merely one of the applied technologies derived from the application of that same scientific knowledge that it generated at the beginning of civilization.

Scientific physicians have legitimate reasons for attempting to identify themselves with mathematics, physics, chemistry and other exact sciences. This attitude is consonant with the Cartesian philosophy which has so profitably guided the development of modern scientific knowledge. But physicians and their patients know intuitively that medicine – human medicine at least – transcends the natural sciences on which it is based. The science of medicine must be supplemented by the art of medicine.

Medicine as an Art

The reduction of medical problems to simplified phenomena amenable to analysis by orthodox scientific methods has yielded an immense harvest of theoretical knowledge and practical applications. Yet there is a widespread feeling that some of the most important medical problems are being neglected. Crude but meaningful expressions of this feeling are found in the common complaint that physicians deal with the disease but neglect the patient and that scientific medicine has lost contact with the human condition.

As if to underscore the failure of scientific medicine to satisfy certain fundamental human needs, the phenomenal development of medical knowledge has been accompanied by a parallel increase in what an English author has recently called 'fringe' medicine. The various forms of faith-healing and of semi-mystical Oriental practices, the drugs and treatments of folklore remedies, and the perennial attempts to solve the problems of modern man by returning to the ways of nature, are but a few of the countless forms of fringe medicine that prosper in all strata of industrialized Western societies. They are not derived from Western medical science and are often incompatible with its teachings.

Whether all forms of fringe medicine are pure deceit or whether some have real merit is irrelevant here. Their popularity points to the need for a kind of medical action not yet embraced by biomedical science. Successful clinicians have always recognized this basic human need and have urged that the science of medicine be supplemented by the 'art' of medicine. What this mysterious art consists of and how it differs from objective scientific knowledge is not easy to discover.

Certainly the physician's sympathy for the human condition is one basic ingredient of the art of medicine. Numerous writings, from Hippocrates on, express how fundamental and long-standing is this need for compassion in the physician. Closely related is another component of the healing art, the physician's ability to inspire confidence and to help his patient make the best of his natural mechanisms of resistance to disease. There often comes a time in the course of disease when the presence of the doctor constitutes by itself an essential element in the patient's recovery. A third part of the art of medicine is the oft-mentioned requirement that the physician understand his patient in terms of the whole man.

Emphasis on the 'whole man' in medical schools became fashionable at the same time that schools of technology began introducing humanistic subjects on their campuses. Engineers and architects, just like physicians, can successfully relate their work to human welfare only to the extent that they are guided by the knowledge of man's fundamental needs and aspirations. Many medical schools are urging their applicants to cultivate humanistic studies in the hope that acquaintance with philosophy, literature, music and the plastic arts will help young physicians gain a better understanding of the human condition. Ironically, the humanities, long regarded by most scientists and technologists as entertaining but otherwise unessential ornaments of life, are now being called in as necessary to the human success of technological civilization.

Like other human beings, physicians and technologists certainly derive cultural benefits from exposure to the broad atmosphere of courses in philosophy, literature and the arts. That their professional activities can be significantly helped by exposure to these disciplines is questionable. While humanists can grasp the universal and eternal aspects of human life, they should not be expected to throw much light on the new problems constantly encountered in the modern world. Modern man, with his endlessly changing environment and ways of life, has to meet challenges for which there are no precedents.

Man feels threatened – and is threatened – by persistent, unavoidable exposure to the stimuli of urban and industrial civilization, and by all the other varied and insulting demands of modern technological society on his fundamental biological nature. What the physician sees, and the problems with which he must deal, find their origins in man's struggle to cope with these constant, ever fluctuating pressures. To a large extent the disorders of the body and the mind are but the expressions of inadequate responses to environmental influences.

Physicians, like technologists, can deal effectively with the problems and needs of human life in the modern world only if they can base their action on a science of man's nature designed to supplement the age-old wisdom transmitted through the humanities.

The Science of Man and Humanism

For several thousand years the humanistic tradition has acquired and transmitted a broad and subtle understanding of the human condition, in happiness and in despair. For three hundred years the biomedical sciences have accumulated an immense number of detailed facts about the human body and mind, in health and in disease. Imposing as they are and complementary as they appear to be, these two aspects of knowledge do not constitute together a true science of man. They do not even form a coherent structure, because the aspects of human biology studied most by scientists have little relevance to the human condition as apprehended by humanists or as expressed by artists.

One often hears that creative artists, humanists and scientists all deal with the same world and differ only in the techniques that they use to recognize and describe reality. Although largely true in the past, probably until the end of the Renaissance, this statement no longer applies. Scientists and humanists are now concerned with entirely different aspects of reality even when they are looking at the same living organism. Stated in an oversimplified form, scientists deal with the material bases of life, whereas humanists and creative artists concentrate on the experience of life.

Biologists tend to focus their professional attention on the structures and mechanisms through which living organisms function and on a few environmental factors that can be measured and manipulated. In the past few decades they have tended to call 'scientific' and 'fundamental' those studies dealing with the elemental structures and reactions common to all forms of life. Of great significance is their habit of speaking of living *things*; usually they feel most at ease when the thing they study is no longer living. Humanists and artists in contrast are little if at all concerned with the fundamental operating structures and mechanisms of living organisms; they want to deal with the experiences of whole men and women responding in all their complexity to the stimuli and challenges of their total environment.[1]

Admittedly, the humanness of man creates problems not definable in scientific terms, and the experience of life is so personal that it does not readily lend itself to experimentation or even observation. Nevertheless, many of man's responses to life situations are amenable to objective study.

Some of man's responses are naturally the direct result of the effects of environmental forces on his body machine. Man responds, however, not as a mechanical assemblage of parts but as a highly integrated organism. Any impinging physico-

1. Although the difference between the natural sciences and the humanities is so profound, the processes involved in the discovery of new scientific facts or in the development of scientific generalizations have much in common with those resulting in the creation of poetry, music or painting. The act of discovery or of creation implies the ability to perceive the external world and to react to it in a fresh manner, uninhibited by the strictures of the past. Whether scientist or artist, the discoverer or creator experiences a sense of joy, wonder and elegance. The similarity in the mechanisms and experiences associated with discovery or creation does not imply similarity in the subject matter or in the products of these activities. In practice, most biological science is irrelevant to the humanist interested in responses and experiences of living man.

chemical or psychic stimulus sets in motion a host of secondary processes with indirect and often delayed effects. Hearing a faint but unexpected noise at night may cause either a rise or a fall in blood pressure; seeing an object that recalls an article of food may stimulate appetite or cause nausea; smelling a perfume may evoke the heat of a summer day or the chill of an autumn evening. The past experience of the person determines the manner of his response to a given stimulus. The primary direct effects of stimuli commonly have little bearing on their ultimate expressions. Each person incorporates the past in his own being. One could almost say that man incarnates history. For this reason, if for none other, a true picture of man cannot come from a study of his components. The past, like the mind, disappears when the organism is taken apart.

Many other difficulties stand in the way of a science of man. Perhaps the greatest of these is that each individual life is made up of unique situations not susceptible to the generalizations of scientific emphasis and terminology. In many ways, however, all men have in common many fundamental traits, and most members of any given culture share a number of experiences, values and modes of thought which make their responses statistically predictable. The science of man could therefore be based on a large body of working assumptions enabling scientists to assess the effect of certain environmental conditions on health and performance.

Since all important responses have multiple determinants, new scientific methods will have to be developed to investigate complex systems in which various factors act simultaneously. Although the study of the complex problems posed by man's responses to new environments will require the participation of many scientific specialities, medicine seems best suited to preside in an architectonic way over the development of a new science of human life. Granted the inescapable limitations of their training in the various specialized sciences, physicians have overwhelming advantages derived from bedside experience; they become familiar through practice with the fundamental needs and potentialities of the human condition. One of the rewards of medical training is a heightened awareness of the complexity and plasticity of man's nature, and some knowledge of the creative way in which most human beings respond to environmental challenges.

The development of methods for studying the responses of the integrated organism would complement the reductionist analysis of structures and mechanisms and enlarge enormously the scope of biomedical sciences. The study of responses is medical biology par excellence since it provides information bearing directly on the well-being of man.

The role of medicine is to help man function well, as long as feasible, and if possible, happily in all his endeavours – whether he is toiling for his daily bread, creating urban civilization, writing a poem or attempting to reach the moon. These examples are not taken at random; they symbolize that medicine relates to all human activities, to the responses of man in the worlds of nature, thought, feeling and technology.

Medicine was, at the beginning of civilization, the mother of sciences, and played a large role in the integration of early cultures. Later it constituted the bridge over which science and humanism maintained some contact. Today it has once more the opportunity of becoming a catalytic force in civilization by pointing to the need, and providing the leadership, for the development of a science of man.

The continued growth of technological civilization, indeed its very survival, requires an enlargement of our understanding of man's nature. Man can function well only when his external environment is in tune with the needs he has inherited from his evolutionary, experiential and social past, and with his aspirations for the future. Because they are concerned with all the various aspects of man's humanness, the biomedical sciences in their highest form are potentially the richest expression of science.

Index

Man and The Cosmos

The Nature of Science Today

Ritchie Calder

That 'science is the everlasting interrogation of Nature by man' is the governing theme of this study by Lord Ritchie-Calder. His aim is to discover 'where science is going', and his survey covers the nature and history of science and the scientific revolution, the dimensions of time and space, and the nature of the universe – both the macrocosmos and the microcosmos. He employs numerous and intriguing pieces of information to illustrate his discussion and shows that it is indeed possible for the layman to gain an insight into the processes of science and its fantastic progression in the second half of the twentieth century.

'... knowledgable and succinct . . . . The book's a splendid read' – *New Scientist* 'This is the best book that Lord Ritchie-Calder has given his readers, and as good as anyone could want for finding out what contemporary science is about' – *The Times Literary Supplement*

Not for sale in the U.S.A. or Canada

More about Penguins
and Pelicans

Penguinews, which appears every month, contains details of all the new books issued by Penguins as they are published. From time to time it is supplemented by *Penguins in Print*, which is a complete list of all books published by Penguins which are in print. (There are well over three thousand of these.)

A specimen copy of *Penguinews* will be sent to you free on request, and you can become a subscriber for the price of the postage. For a year's issues (including the complete lists) please send 4s. if you live in the United Kingdom, or 8s. if you live elsewhere. Just write to Dept EP, Penguin Books Ltd, Harmondsworth, Middlesex, enclosing a cheque or postal order, and your name will be added to the mailing list.

Another Pelican book is described on the following page.

Note: *Penguinews* and *Penguins in Print* are not available in the U.S.A. or Canada